healthcare

Special Issue Reprint

Pharmacy Practice and Administration 2.0

Edited by
Georges Adunlin

mdpi.com/journal/healthcare

MDPI

Pharmacy Practice and Administration 2.0

Pharmacy Practice and Administration 2.0

Editor

Georges Adunlin

MDPI

Basel • Beijing • Wuhan • Barcelona • Belgrade • Novi Sad • Cluj • Manchester

Editor
Georges Adunlin
Department of Pharmaceutical,
Social and Administrative Sciences
Samford University
Birmingham
United States

Editorial Office
MDPI
St. Alban-Anlage 66
4052 Basel, Switzerland

This is a reprint of articles from the Special Issue published online in the open access journal *Healthcare* (ISSN 2227-9032) (available at: www.mdpi.com/journal/healthcare/special_issues/Pharmacy_Practice_Administration_2).

For citation purposes, cite each article independently as indicated on the article page online and as indicated below:

Lastname, A.A.; Lastname, B.B. Article Title. *Journal Name* **Year**, *Volume Number*, Page Range.

ISBN 978-3-7258-0566-2 (Hbk)
ISBN 978-3-7258-0565-5 (PDF)
doi.org/10.3390/books978-3-7258-0565-5

Contents

About the Editor

Georges Adunlin

Georges Adunlin, PhD, MA, MSEd, is an Associate Professor at Samford University, McWhorter School of Pharmacy. His research uses pharmacoeconomic, economic, and epidemiologic methodologies to analyze complex datasets. Specifically, Dr. Adunlin's research involves issues related to advances in cancer care technologies, such as emerging treatments and diagnostics, and how these advances in technologies impact different cancer outcomes and experiences such as access, quality of care, cost of care, and health disparities. He has a passion for teaching and learning and strives to create excellent instructional outcomes by bringing together pedagogical expertise, innovative classroom practices, and student support for the application of learning. Dr. Adunlin's scholarship of Teaching and Learning focuses on educational technology and assessment strategies.

healthcare

MDPI

Article

Impact of Sertraline, Fluoxetine, and Escitalopram on Psychological Distress among United States Adult Outpatients with a Major Depressive Disorder

Kwame Adjei [1], Georges Adunlin [2] and Askal Ayalew Ali [1,*]

[1] Department of Economic, Social and Administrative Pharmacy, Florida Agricultural and Mechanical University, Tallahassee, FL 32307, USA
[2] Department of Pharmaceutical, Social and Administrative Sciences, Samford University, Birmingham, AL 35229, USA
* Correspondence: askal.ali@famu.edu; Tel.: +1-850-599-3082

Abstract: How impactful is the use of Sertraline, Fluoxetine, and Escitalopram monotherapy on psychological distress among adults with depression in the real world? Selective serotonin reuptake inhibitors (SSRIs) are the most commonly prescribed antidepressants. Medical Expenditure Panel Survey (MEPS) longitudinal data files from 1 January 2012 to 31 December 2019 (panel 17–23) were used to assess the effects of Sertraline, Fluoxetine and Escitalopram on psychological distress among adult outpatients diagnosed with a major depressive disorder. Participants aged 20–80 years without comorbidities, who initiated antidepressants only at rounds 2 and 3 of each panel, were included. The impact of the medicines on psychological distress was assessed using changes in Kessler Index (K6) scores, which were measured only in rounds 2 and 4 of each panel. Multinomial logistic regression was conducted using the changes in the K6 scores as a dependent variable. A total of 589 participants were included in the study. Overall, 90.79% of the study participants on monotherapy antidepressants reported improved levels of psychological distress. Fluoxetine had the highest improvement rate of 91.87%, followed by Escitalopram (90.38%) and Sertraline (90.27%). The findings on the comparative effectiveness of the three medications were statistically insignificant. Sertraline, Fluoxetine, and Escitalopram were shown to be effective among adult patients suffering from major depressive disorders without comorbid conditions.

Keywords: Sertraline; Fluoxetine; Escitalopram; psychological distress; monotherapy; Kessler Index; major depressive disorder; serotonin transporter; antidepressants

Citation: Adjei, K.; Adunlin, G.; Ali, A.A. Impact of Sertraline, Fluoxetine, and Escitalopram on Psychological Distress among United States Adult Outpatients with a Major Depressive Disorder. *Healthcare* **2023**, *11*, 740. https://doi.org/10.3390/healthcare11050740

Academic Editor: Axel Steiger

Received: 31 January 2023
Revised: 25 February 2023
Accepted: 2 March 2023
Published: 3 March 2023

1. Introduction

Approximately 15 million physician office visits with depressive disorders as the primary diagnosis were recorded in 2019 [1]. An estimated 21 million adults and 4.1 million adolescents aged 12 to 17 in the USA in 2017 had at least one major depressive episode, representing 8.4% and 17% of the USA population, respectively [2]. According to the World Health Organization, depression is ranked as the most significant cause of disability worldwide and contributes heavily to the global disease burden [3]. Depression is the major contributing factor to suicide and ischemic heart disease [4].

"According to the Global Burden of Disease study, major depressive disorder was recorded as the mental health disorder with the highest economic burden accounting for 2.7 million disability-adjusted life years in 2016" [5]. In 2018, the economic burden of depression was estimated at USD 326 billion, representing an increase of 37.9% between 2010 and 2018 [6]. "The Center for Disease Control emphasizes that over the past two decades, the use of antidepressants has experienced tremendous growth, making them one of the most expensive and third most prescribed drugs in the USA" [7].

First-generation antidepressants, such as tricyclic antidepressants and monoamine oxidase inhibitors, used to be the main treatment for depression, but they are no longer preferred in many clinics due to their serious side effects, such as orthostatic hypotension and insomnia [8–10]. Second-generation antidepressants, including selective serotonin reuptake inhibitors (SSRIs), serotonin and norepinephrine reuptake inhibitors (SNRIs), and dopamine reuptake inhibitors, have fewer side effects than first-generation antidepressants [11]. Fluoxetine and Sertraline were among the first SSRIs approved for depression treatment in the 1990s, and Escitalopram was introduced in 2003 [12]. Although the different classes of second-generation antidepressants have similar effectiveness on quality of life, they differ in their pharmacokinetics, pharmacodynamics, and side effects, which may impact treatment selection [13]. Fluoxetine has a lower specificity of serotonin transporter (SERT) than other SSRIs, but a better binding specificity than tricyclic antidepressants and monoamine oxidase inhibitors [14,15]. Fluoxetine can lead to weight loss, agitation, and anxiety; Sertraline is associated with a higher incidence of diarrhea; and Escitalopram has a higher likelihood than other SSRIs of causing QT prolongation [16–18].

In clinical practice, second-generation antidepressants are prescribed for many conditions other than depression, such as anxiety, sleeping disorders, psychosis, and neuropathic pain [19]. "Sertraline is currently approved for major depressive disorder, obsessive-compulsive disorder, panic disorder, post-traumatic stress disorder, seasonal affective disorder, and premenstrual dysphoric disorder" [14]. Escitalopram is also used in the management of generalized anxiety disorder, while Fluoxetine is used in the treatment of premenstrual dysphoric disorder [14]. The choice of antidepressants is influenced by drug profiles, physician characteristics, patient characteristics, and other factors such as comorbidities [20,21].

"Psychological distress refers to non-specific symptoms of stress, anxiety, and depression. High levels of psychological distress are indicative of impaired mental health and may reflect common mental disorders, like depressive and anxiety disorders" [22]. Research has shown that individuals with depression often experience high levels of psychological distress in various areas of life, which leads to a decline in physical, emotional, and social functioning [23]. Physical symptoms of depression, such as fatigue and changes in appetite and sleep patterns, can negatively impact an individual's ability to engage in physical activity and maintain good physical health [23,24]. Emotional symptoms, such as feelings of sadness and hopelessness, can lead to difficulty in maintaining personal relationships and a lack of interest in activities. Social functioning may also be affected, as individuals with depression may withdraw from social interactions and have difficulty in forming and maintaining relationships [23].

In addition to the negative impact of psychological distress, depression also increases the risk of various physical health problems, such as cardiovascular disease, diabetes, and obesity which can be attributed to unhealthy coping mechanisms such as overeating, lack of physical activity, and substance abuse [24,25]. It is important for individuals with depression to receive appropriate treatment and support to improve their overall well-being and functioning.

There are widely used survey instruments for measuring psychological distress in people with depression, such as the Patient Health Questionnaire-9 (PHQ-9), the Beck Depression Inventory (BDI), and the Kessler Psychological Distress Scale (K6). "The PHQ-9 is a self-administered questionnaire that assesses the presence and severity of depressive symptoms over the past two weeks, consisting of nine items rated on a four-point Likert scale" [26]. The BDI is a 21-item self-report inventory that measures the presence and severity of depression symptoms over the past two weeks, assessing symptoms such as sadness, hopelessness, and self-esteem, each rated on a four-point Likert scale [27]. The K6 is a brief, self-administered questionnaire that assesses symptoms of non-specific psychological distress over the past 30 days, consisting of six items rated on a five-point Likert scale. A score of 13 or higher on the K6 is considered to indicate clinically significant psychological distress [28].

The K6 is a reliable and valid measure of psychological distress among patients with depression. It has good test–retest reliability, with a correlation coefficient of 0.8, and strong concurrent validity, as it correlates well with other measures of depression and anxiety and is able to discriminate between patients with depression and those without depression [28,29].

Over 40% of depression patients fail to improve with conventional treatment, which involves using a single antidepressant agent at a prescribed dose and duration [30–33]. In spite of the considerable amount of data available on the clinical efficacy of second-generation antidepressants, there remains insufficient evidence on the real-world impact of the most widely prescribed second-generation antidepressants on patient-reported outcomes.

This study evaluated the effectiveness of the most commonly prescribed antidepressants, Sertraline, Fluoxetine and Escitalopram, on psychological distress among various subgroup populations based on age, race, and sex using a nationally representative sample in the United States.

2. Materials and Methods

2.1. Data Source

The current retrospective longitudinal study was conducted to examine the effectiveness of Sertraline, Fluoxetine, and Escitalopram monotherapy on psychological distress as a patient-reported outcome among the non-institutionalized US population using the Medical Expenditure Panel Survey (MEPS). The MEPS data used in this study spanned the period 1 January 2012 to 31 December 2019 (panel 17 to panel 23) [34].

The MEPS is a nationally representative estimate of health care use, expenditure, sources of payment, health insurance coverage, and demographic characteristics, additionally providing data on respondents' health status, employment, access to care, and satisfaction with healthcare [34]. "The National Health Interview Survey (NHIS) uses a stratified, multistage probability cluster sampling design which provides a nationally representative sample of the U.S. civilian, non-institutionalized population" [34]. "A computer assisted personal interviewing (CAPI) technology is used to collect information about each household member and the information collected for a sampled household is reported by a single household respondent. Verification of patient's reports are conducted through a survey response from their healthcare providers and contacting the pharmacies where the participants reported of filling their prescribed medicines" [34,35]. The panel design of the survey comprises five rounds of interviews covering two full calendar years (Figure 1).

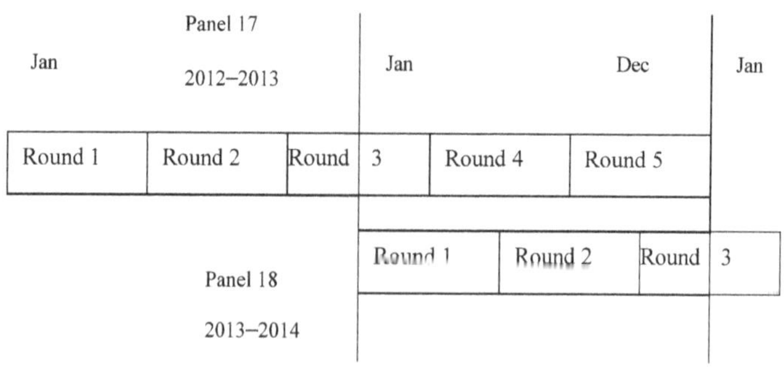

Figure 1. Adopted from MEPS AHRQ panel design [34].

Depression was defined as a major depressive episode that affects mood, behavior, and overall health, causing prolonged feelings of sadness, emptiness, or hopelessness and loss of interest in activities that were once enjoyed [35]. Antidepressant monotherapy was defined as patients taking a single antidepressant agent to treat a major depressive disorder. All respondents who were identified as having depression in the 2012–2019 MEPS database, were aged over 19 years, and taking a single agent of Sertraline, Fluoxetine or Escitalopram, were included in the study. To appreciate the effects of the medicine on changes in depressive symptoms during the study, only participants who started taking antidepressants at round 2 and round 3 of the panel were included in the study. The "purchrd" variable was used to select participants from various rounds of the panel. The rationale was to compare the baseline depressive symptoms of the participants from the time they started taking the medications with their symptoms after they had been taking them for roughly a year (in round 4). This will enable us gain insights into the effects of the medicine on the change in depressive symptoms during the study. Patients who purchased medicine before or at the beginning of rounds 1, 4, and 5 of the panel were excluded from the study. Patients who were taking combination therapy were excluded from the study. Patients who had comorbid conditions were also excluded from the study. Respondents with missing responses on the dependent variable (K6 scores) were excluded from the analysis.

2.2. Study Design

The MEPS HC medical condition file was used to identify individuals with depression. The MEPS medical condition file contains information on the observation of each self-reported medical condition that a respondent experienced during the data collection year. Medical conditions reported by participants were recorded by interviews and coded to fully specified ICD-10-CM and ICD-9-CM codes. Depression was identified using ICD-9-code 296, 311, and ICD-10-code F32 [34].

Patients taking antidepressants were identified using the prescribed medicines file (Figure 2). The most commonly used antidepressants, Fluoxetine, Escitalopram, and Sertraline, were identified using "rxname" and "rxdrgnam" variables from the prescribed medicines file [34].

The patients' demographic characteristics were identified from the patient characteristic file. In this study, we included age, race, and gender.

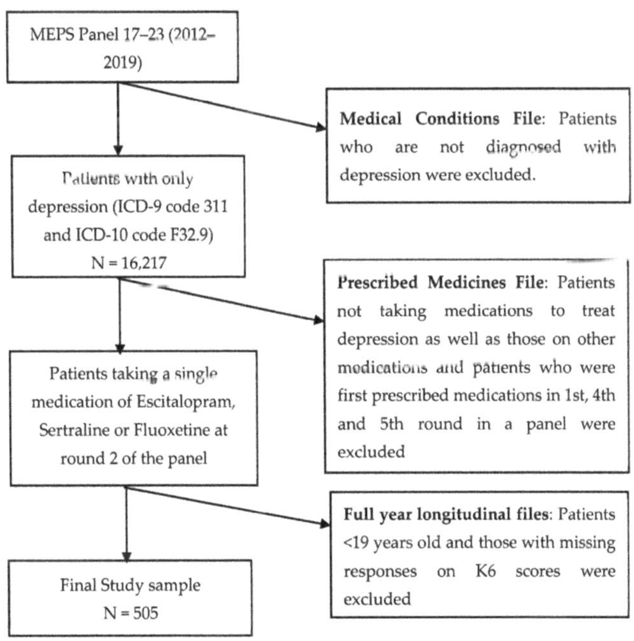

Figure 2. Flowchart of study cohort [28,34].

2.3. Outcome Measures

The effect of the medicines on psychological distress was assessed using the Kessler Index (K6) scores. The Kessler Index (K6) scores measure individuals' non-specific psychological distress in the past 30 days [28]. The scale consists of six items, each rated on a five-point Likert scale (from "none of the time" to "all of the time") [28]. Supplementary S1.

The longitudinal data files in the MEPS contain K6 scores. These scores are measured in rounds 2 and 4 of a panel and are roughly a year apart [36]. Previously reported cut off-points in the literature were used to stratify K6 scores into no/low psychological distress (0–6), mild–moderate psychological distress (7–12), and severe distress (13–24) [28].

In this study, regarding changes in the baseline K6 score (that is round 2–round 4), 1–24 was identified as improved, whereas a change in the K6 score of 0 was classified as unchanged, and when a change in the baseline K6 score ranged from −1 to −24, it was classified as having declined.

2.4. Statistical Analysis

Descriptive statistics were used to describe the population according to their socio-demographic characteristics. All statistical values were considered significant at a level of significance of $p \leq 0.05$. The dependent variable, namely the difference in K6 scores, was categorized using 1–24 as "improved", −1–−24 as "declined" and 0 as "unchanged". A multinomial logistic regression model was built to determine the effect of the independent variables on the above-mentioned dependent variable. Demographic variables such as race, gender, and age were controlled in the regression analysis. Statistical analysis was conducted using STATA software (version 15.1).

3. Results

Demographic Characteristics of Study Population

Table 1 shows the demographic characteristics of the study population for each antidepressant. Among the three antidepressants used in the analysis, Sertraline was the most utilized medication among the study population (N = 251, 42.61%) followed by Fluoxetine (N = 185, 31.41%). Most of the study population were females (N = 417), representing 70.5% of the total study sample. Among different races, non-Hispanic whites were the highest users (N = 489, 83.02%) of the three SSRIs, with American Indians being the lowest users (N = 9, 1.53%) of the three SSRIs. Most of the study population was within the 40–59 age group (N = 244, 38.54%).

Table 1. Demographic characteristics of study participants on the various antidepressants.

Characteristics	Escitalopram N (%)	Sertraline N (%)	Fluoxetine N (%)
Total	153 (25.98)	251 (42.61)	185 (31.41)
Gender			
Male	34 (22)	73 (29)	67 (36)
Female	119 (78)	178 (71)	118 (64)
Age			
20–39	48 (31.2)	80 (31.9)	54 (29.0)
40–59	65 (42.5)	99 (39.6)	[illegible] (40.1)
60–80	40 (26.2)	72 (28.5)	51 (27.9)
Race			
White	129 (84.31)	205 (81.67)	155 (83.78)
Black	11 (7.19)	29 (11.55)	15 (8.11)
American Indian	1 (0.65)	5 (1.99)	3 (1.62)
Asian	4 (2.61)	4 (1.59)	7 (3.78)
Multi-race	8 (5.23)	8 (3.19)	5 (2.70)

Table 2 shows the percentage of patients on Sertraline, Fluoxetine, and Escitalopram who showed improvement, no change, or decline in Kessler 6 scores. The majority of the patients (N = 467, 92.48%) were in the improved group, regardless of which of the three medications they were taking. Fluoxetine had the highest improvement rate of 94.27%, compared with Sertraline, which had an improvement rate of 91.96%, and Escitalopram, which had an improvement rate of 91.13%.

Table 2. Percentage of individuals showing a change in K6 scores based on Fluoxetine, Escitalopram, Sertraline.

Second-Generation Antidepressants	Improved N (%) 467 (92.48)	Unchanged N (%) 31 (6.14)	Declined N (%) 7 (1.39)
Fluoxetine	148 (94.27)	6 (3.82)	3 (1.91)
Escitalopram	113 (91.13)	10 (8.06)	1 (0.81)
Sertraline	206 (91.96)	15 (6.70)	3 (1.34)

Table 3 shows the multinomial logistic regression results for changes in the Kessler Index scores among patients taking Sertraline, Fluoxetine, or Escitalopram monotherapy. A total of 84 participants with missing responses on the Kessler Index score were excluded, resulting in 505 participants being included in the regression analysis. Participants in the unchanged K6 category were used as references to predict improvement in psychological distress for users on the three SSRIs. Moreover, participants taking Fluoxetine were treated as the reference group among the three medications. Among the various age groups, participants aged between 20 and 39 years were used as the reference group, while non-Hispanic whites were used as the reference for race. In comparison with the participants taking Fluoxetine, the results did not show any statistical difference between participants taking Escitalopram (OR = 0.2823, 95% CI, 0.0209–3.812; $p = 0.34$) and those taking Sertraline (OR = 0.45, 95% CI, 0.06–3.3249; $p = 0.43$).

Table 3. Multinomial logistic regression to predict improvement in K6 scores among SSRIs users.

Category Ref: Unchanged	Improvement Rate		Declined Rate	
	OR (95% CI)	*p*-Value	OR (95% CI)	*p*-Value
Drug ref: Fluoxetine				
Escitalopram	0.2823 (0.0209–3.812)	0.340	0.4269 (0.1209–1.5067)	0.185
Sertraline	0.4500 (0.06–3.3249)	0.433	1.088 (0.2885–4.1027)	0.901
Sex: Female				
Male	0.839 (0.466–1.212)	0.530	0.605 (0.081–1.129)	0.15
Age ref: 20–39				
40–59	0.9911 (0.0998–9.839)	0.994	1.8426 (0.5442–6.2379)	0.325
60–80	0.6620 (0.0553–7.922)	0.744	0.9330 (0.2930–2.9701)	0.906
Race ref: White				
Black	33.304 (2.671–415.19)	0.007	8.7937 (1.099–70.3069)	0.040
American Indian	6.22 (0.3324–116.39)	0.221	1.50 (1.35–1.66)	0.00
Asian	5.31 (0.2243–125.79)	0.300	0.5961 (0.0680–5.1633)	0.638
Multi-race	1.80 (0.356–9.095)	0.476	4.43 (3.88–4.98)	0.00

4. Discussion

Patients with a major depressive disorder usually have deteriorating mental health that affects the physical and social aspects of their lives. The primary aim of this study was to assess the effects of Sertraline, Fluoxetine, and Escitalopram on psychological distress using changes in Kessler Index 6 scores among adult outpatients diagnosed with one major depressive disorder.

The study sample was characterized by over 70% women, which corresponds with other studies that show that women are more likely than men to experience more depression. Females are also more likely than men to report to a mental health facility or seek medical attention [37,38]. In addition, the increased prevalence of depression correlates with hormonal changes in women, particularly during puberty, before menstruation, following pregnancy, and at perimenopause, suggesting that female hormonal fluctuations may trigger depression [39,40].

The majority of the study population were non-Hispanic whites. Similar racial/ethnic differences in antidepressant use are observed in the treatment of depression [41]. It has also been reported that factors such as racial/ethnic variation in mental health services and availability, treatment acceptability, and educational factors play a role in the prevalence of depression and antidepressant use among races [42]. The 40–59 age group was the highest population taking antidepressant monotherapy, representing over 38% of the study sample. On the contrary, recent studies have shown that young adults aged 18–29 have a higher prevalence of depression than older adults [43,44]. In part, the COVID-19 pandemic has been identified to have played a major role in the increase in the prevalence of depression among young adults [30–32]. Young adults have suffered from higher levels of depression and anxiety than older adults throughout the pandemic [45]. According to the Centers for Disease Control and Prevention's (CDC) Household Pulse Survey, 36% of 18–29-year-olds had symptoms of depression in early May 2021, compared to 22% of those aged 40–49 and 15% of those aged 50–59 [45].

The descriptive statistics showed that 94.27% of the study participants taking Fluoxetine had experienced an improvement in their psychological distress after one year on the medication, followed by Sertraline (91.96%) and Escitalopram (91.13%). The overall improvement rate of 92.48% among the study sample indicates only that selective serotonin reuptake inhibitor medication effectively improves patient-reported outcomes, specifically psychological distress, over one year of taking the medication. In a similar study, the majority of the participants taking either first- or second-generation antidepressant monotherapy remained in the unchanged category after round 4 [36]. The authors explained that the medications might have elicited desirable responses resulting in patients having controlled depressive symptoms even at the time of the initial measure (round 2 of the panel) of psychological distress [37].

The current study compared the impact of Fluoxetine, Sertraline, and Escitalopram on patient-reported outcomes and psychological distress using changes in the Kessler 6 score. In our comparison with Fluoxetine as a reference drug, there was no statistical difference observed between the effect of Sertraline (OR = 0.45, 95% CI, 0.06–3.3249; p = 0.43), and Escitalopram (OR = 0.2823, 95% CI, 0.0209–3.812; p = 0.34) on psychological distress. Currently, there is insufficient data on evaluating the effectiveness of these commonly prescribed antidepressants using changes in the Kessler 6 score as a patient-reported outcome. A similar study on changes in the Kessler Index 6 score showed no significant difference between patients using monotherapy and those using add-on/switch therapy [36]. However, comparing our results to a meta-analysis involving 24,595 participants in 111 studies on the efficacy and acceptability of 12 antidepressants, Escitalopram, Sertraline, and Fluoxetine were found to have superior efficacy than the SNRIs in the meta-analysis [46]. With Fluoxetine as a reference compound, both Escitalopram and Sertraline had a significantly higher efficacy rate than Fluoxetine. However, they concluded that Sertraline may be preferable because of the balance between its efficacy and its tolerability [46,47]. In these studies, the treatment effect was measured using another instrument variable, changes in the baseline Montgomery–Asberg Depression Rating Scale (MADRS) total score.

The strength of this study was that a retrospective longitudinal database was used with a nationally representative sample. Due to the structure of the Medical Expenditure Panel Survey (MEPS), we were able to assess the outcome of the medications on psychological distress over time points approximately one year apart (from round 2 to round 4). This gives adequate time to elicit rich data on the long-term effect of the medications on the participants, which is essential for a chronic disease with a high relapse rate, such as depression. However, there were limitations to the study. This study focused on patients with a major depressive disorder without any comorbidities. This limits the generalizability of the results. The study is susceptible to response bias, as the information is self-reported by respondents and cannot therefore always be considered reliable. Moreover, this study could not adjust for the type and severity of depression, illness duration, side effects, and medication adherence, due to the structure of the MEPS. Additionally, this study could not account for the specific dose and titration of the medication, due to the nature of the MEPS, which does not provide dose-related information on the medications. We assumed that patients were prescribed the standard dose of the medications: Escitalopram 10–20 mg once a day [48], Sertraline 150–200 mg daily [49], and Fluoxetine 20–60 mg per day [50]. A future study could focus on examining the real-world impacts of these most widely prescribed antidepressants together with newly approved antidepressants, taking into account medication adherence, the tolerability of the medications, and the type and severity of depression. Due to insufficient evidence on the real-world impacts of selective serotonin reuptake inhibitors among depressed patients, this study adds to the evidence available to inform clinicians on the effect of the long-term use of selective serotonin reuptake inhibitors on patient-reported outcomes among patients with chronic depression. This study can also serve as a guide for researchers in this area, who can focus on the use of second-generation antidepressant monotherapy and dual-therapy antidepressants among patients with severe depression using real-world data.

5. Conclusions

Based on the descriptive statistics, all the medications effectively improve the rate of psychological distress among adult patients suffering from major depressive disorders without comorbid conditions. Moreover, no significant difference in the improvement rate of psychological distress for the participants was observed in our comparison of the three selective serotonin reuptake inhibitors. In addition to taking the effectiveness of the medications into account, it is imperative that clinicians consider patients' preferences and tolerability toward specific antidepressant medications in their prescribing decisions.

Supplementary Materials: The following supporting information can be downloaded at: https://www.mdpi.com/article/10.3390/healthcare11050740/s1, S1: Kessler Index (K6) score.

Author Contributions: Conceptualization K.A.; Methodology: all authors; Formal analysis: all authors; Writing—Original Draft Preparation: K.A.; Writing—Review & Editing: A.A.A. and G.A.; Visualization: all authors; Supervision: A.A.A. and G.A.; Project Administration: A.A.A. and G.A. All authors have read and agreed to the published version of the manuscript.

Funding: This research received no external funding.

Institutional Review Board Statement: Ethical review and approval were waived for this study since the study utilized data collected by another institution, the Medical Expenditure Panel Survey. Therefore, we did not have any contact with or identification on the study participants.

Informed Consent Statement: Not applicable.

Data Availability Statement: Publicly available datasets were analyzed in this study. This data can be found here: https://www.meps.ahrq.gov/mepsweb/ (accessed on 21 September 2021).

Acknowledgments: We would like to acknowledge Florida A&M University for its overall support. The authors acknowledge Title III for its financial assistance.

Conflicts of Interest: The authors declare no conflict of interest.

References

1. Santo, L.; Kang, K. National Hospital Ambulatory Medical Care Survey: 2019 National Summary Tables. 20 January 2023. Available online: https://stacks.cdc.gov/view/cdc/123251 (accessed on 21 February 2023).
2. NIMH » Major Depression. The National Institute of Mental Health Information Resource Center. 2020. Available online: https://www.nimh.nih.gov/health/statistics/major-depression#part_2631 (accessed on 29 September 2021).
3. Depression. 13 September 2021. Available online: https://www.who.int/news-room/fact-sheets/detail/depression (accessed on 28 November 2021).

4. Shah, A.J. Depression and History of Attempted Suicide as Risk Factors for Heart Disease Mortality in Young Individuals. *Arch. Gen. Psychiatry* **2011**, *68*, 1135–1142. [CrossRef]
5. Greenberg, P.E.; Fournier, A.-A.; Sisitsky, T.; Pike, C.T.; Kessler, R.C. The Economic Burden of Adults with Major Depressive Disorder in the United States (2005 and 2010). *J. Clin. Psychiatry* **2015**, *76*, 155–162. [CrossRef] [PubMed]
6. Greenberg, P.E.; Fournier, A.-A.; Sisitsky, T.; Simes, M.; Berman, R.; Koenigsberg, S.H.; Kessler, R.C. The Economic Burden of Adults with Major Depressive Disorder in the United States (2010 and 2018). *Pharmacoeconomics* **2021**, *39*, 653–665. [CrossRef] [PubMed]
7. Antidepressant Use among Persons Aged 12 and Over: United States, 2011–2014. Centers for Disease Control and Prevention. August 2017. Available online: https://www.cdc.gov/nchs/products/databriefs/db283.htm (accessed on 11 October 2021).
8. Thaler, K.; Gartlehner, G.; Hansen, R.; Morgan, L.; Lux, L.; Van Noord, M.; Mager, U.; Gaynes, B.; Thieda, P.; Strobelberger, M.; et al. The comparative efficacy of second-generation antidepressants for the accompanying symptoms of depression: A systematic review. *Eur. Psychiatry* **2011**, *26*, 697. [CrossRef]
9. Song, F.; Freemantle, N.; Sheldon, T.A.; House, A.; Watson, P.; Long, A.; Mason, J. Selective serotonin reuptake inhibitors: Meta-analysis of efficacy and acceptability. *BMJ* **1993**, *306*, 683–687. [CrossRef] [PubMed]
10. Montgomery, S.A.; Henry, J.; McDonald, G.; Dinan, T.; Lader, M.; Hindmarch, I.; Clare, A.; Nutt, D. Selective serotonin reuptake inhibitors. *Int. Clin. Psychopharmacol.* **1994**, *9*, 47–54. [CrossRef]
11. Ferguson, J.M. SSRI Antidepressant Medications. *Prim. Care Companion J. Clin. Psychiatry* **2001**, *3*, 22–27. [CrossRef]
12. Sanchez, C.; Reines, E.H.; Montgomery, S.A. A comparative review of escitalopram, paroxetine, and sertraline. *Int. Clin. Psychopharmacol.* **2014**, *29*, 185–196. [CrossRef] [PubMed]
13. Sheridan, S.D.A. Second-Generation Antidepressants for Depression in Adults. Implementing AHRQ Effective Health Care Reviews-American Family Physician. 15 November 2013. Available online: https://www.aafp.org/afp/2013/1115/p687.html#afp20131115p687-b1 (accessed on 11 October 2021).
14. Edinoff, A.; Akuly, H.; Hanna, T.; Ochoa, C.; Patti, S.; Ghaffar, Y.; Kaye, A.; Viswanath, O.; Urits, I.; Boyer, A.; et al. Selective Serotonin Reuptake Inhibitors and Adverse Effects: A Narrative Review. *Neurol. Int.* **2021**, *13*, 387–401. [CrossRef]
15. Bymaster, F.P.; Zhang, W.; Carter, P.A.; Shaw, J.; Chernet, E.; Phebus, L.; Wong, D.T.; Perry, K.W. Fluoxetine, but not other selective serotonin uptake inhibitors, increases norepinephrine and dopamine extracellular levels in prefrontal cortex. *Psychopharmacology* **2002**, *160*, 353–361. [CrossRef]
16. Marken, P.A.; Munro, J.S. Selecting a Selective Serotonin Reuptake Inhibitor. *Prim. Care Companion J. Clin. Psychiatry* **2000**, *2*, 205–210. [CrossRef]
17. Lam, R. Antidepressants and QTc prolongation. *J. Psychiatry Neurosci.* **2013**, *38*, E5–E6. [CrossRef]
18. Hashimoto, K. Sigma-1 Receptors and Selective Serotonin Reuptake Inhibitors: Clinical Implications of their Relationship. *Central Nerv. Syst. Agents Med. Chem.* **2009**, *9*, 197–204. [CrossRef]
19. Noordam, R.; Aarts, N.; Verhamme, K.M.; Sturkenboom, M.C.M.; Stricker, B.H.; Visser, L.E. Prescription and indication trends of antidepressant drugs in the Netherlands between 1996 and 2012: A dynamic population-based study. *Eur. J. Clin. Pharmacol.* **2015**, *71*, 369–375. [CrossRef] [PubMed]
20. Forns, J.; Pottegård, A.; Reinders, T.; Poblador-Plou, B.; Morros, R.; Brandt, L.; Cainzos-Achirica, M.; Hellfritzsch, M.; Schink, T.; Prados-Torres, A.; et al. Antidepressant use in Denmark, Germany, Spain, and Sweden between 2009 and 2014: Incidence and comorbidities of antidepressant initiators. *J. Affect. Disord.* **2019**, *249*, 242–252. [CrossRef] [PubMed]
21. Haro, J.M.; Lamy, F.-X.; Jönsson, B.; Knapp, M.; Brignone, M.; Caillou, H.; Chalem, Y.; Hammer-Helmich, L.; Rive, B.; Saragoussi, D. Characteristics of patients with depression initiating or switching antidepressant treatment: Baseline analyses of the PERFORM cohort study. *BMC Psychiatry* **2018**, *18*, 80. [CrossRef]
22. Cuijpers, P.; Smits, N.; Donker, T.; Have, M.T.; de Graaf, R. Screening for mood and anxiety disorders with the five-item, the three-item, and the two-item Mental Health Inventory. *Psychiatry Res.* **2009**, *168*, 250–255. [CrossRef] [PubMed]
23. Viertiö, S.; Kiviruusu, O.; Piirtola, M.; Kaprio, J.; Korhonen, T.; Marttunen, M.; Suvisaari, J. Factors contributing to psychological distress in the working population, with a special reference to gender difference. *BMC Public Health* **2021**, *21*, 611. [CrossRef]
24. Mauramo, E.; Lahti, J.; Lallukka, T.; Lahelma, E.; Pietiläinen, O.; Rahkonen, O. Changes in common mental disorders and diagnosis-specific sickness absence: A register-linkage follow-up study among Finnish municipal employees. *Occup. Environ. Med.* **2019**, *76*, [illegible]. [CrossRef]
25. Jena, B.N.; Kalra, S.; Yeravdekar, R. Emotional and psychological needs of people with diabetes. *Indian J. Endocrinol. Metab.* **2018**, *22*, 696–704. [CrossRef]
26. Kroenke, K.; Spitzer, R.L.; Williams, J.B.W.; Löwe, B. The Patient Health Questionnaire Somatic, Anxiety, and Depressive Symptom Scales: A systematic review. *Gen. Hosp. Psychiatry* **2010**, *32*, 345–359. [CrossRef] [PubMed]
27. Beck, A.T.; Steer, R.A.; Ball, R.; Ranieri, W.F. Comparison of Beck Depression Inventories-IA and-II in Psychiatric Outpatients. *J. Pers. Assess.* **1996**, *67*, 588–597. [CrossRef] [PubMed]
28. Kang, Y.-K.; Guo, W.-J.; Xu, H.; Chen, Y.-H.; Li, X.-J.; Tan, Z.-P.; Li, N.; Gesang, Z.-R.; Wang, Y.-M.; Liu, C.-B.; et al. The 6-item Kessler psychological distress scale to survey serious mental illness among Chinese undergraduates: Psychometric properties and prevalence estimate. *Compr. Psychiatry* **2015**, *63*, 105–112. [CrossRef]

29. Andersen, L.S.; Grimsrud, A.; Myer, L.; Williams, D.R.; Stein, D.J.; Seedat, S. The psychometric properties of the K10 and K6 scales in screening for mood and anxiety disorders in the South African Stress and Health study. *Int. J. Methods Psychiatr. Res.* **2011**, *20*, 215–223. [CrossRef] [PubMed]
30. Shelton, R.C.; Tollefson, G.D.; Tohen, M.; Stahl, S.; Gannon, K.S.; Jacobs, T.G.; Buras, W.R.; Bymaster, F.P.; Zhang, W.; Spencer, K.A.; et al. A Novel Augmentation Strategy for Treating Resistant Major Depression. *Am. J. Psychiatry* **2001**, *158*, 131–134. [CrossRef]
31. Rush, A.J.; Kraemer, H.C.; Sackeim, H.A.; Fava, M.; Trivedi, M.H.; Frank, E.; Ninan, P.T.; Thase, M.E.; Gelenberg, A.J.; Kupfer, D.J.; et al. Report by the ACNP Task Force on Response and Remission in Major Depressive Disorder. *Neuropsychopharmacology* **2006**, *31*, 1841–1853. [CrossRef]
32. Fava, M.; Davidson, K.G. Definition and epidemiology of treatment-resistant depression. *Psychiatr. Clin. N. Am.* **1996**, *19*, 179–200. [CrossRef]
33. Papakostas, G.I.; Shelton, R.C.; Smith, J.; Fava, M. Augmentation of Antidepressants with Atypical Antipsychotic Medications for Treatment-Resistant Major Depressive Disorder: A meta-analysis. *J. Clin. Psychiatry* **2007**, *68*, 826–831. [CrossRef]
34. Methodology Report #24: Estimation Procedures for the 2007 Medical Expenditure Panel Survey Household Component. (n.d.). Available online: https://meps.ahrq.gov/data_files/publications/mr24/mr24.shtml (accessed on 28 September 2021).
35. What Is Depression? (n.d.). American Psychiatry Association. Available online: https://www.psychiatry.org/patients-families/depression/what-is-depression (accessed on 1 November 2021).
36. Shah, D.; Vaidya, V.; Patel, A.; Borovicka, M.; Goodman, M.-H. Assessment of health-related quality of life, mental health status and psychological distress based on the type of pharmacotherapy used among patients with depression. *Qual. Life Res.* **2016**, *26*, 969–980. [CrossRef]
37. Ford, D.E.; Erlinger, T.P. Depression and C-Reactive Protein in US Adults. *Arch. Intern. Med.* **2004**, *164*, 1010–1014. [CrossRef]
38. Salk, R.H.; Hyde, J.S.; Abramson, L.Y. Gender differences in depression in representative national samples: Meta-analyses of diagnoses and symptoms. *Psychol. Bull.* **2017**, *143*, 783–822. [CrossRef] [PubMed]
39. Albert, P.R. Why is depression more prevalent in women? *J. Psychiatry Neurosci.* **2015**, *40*, 219–221. [CrossRef]
40. Bartels, M.; Cacioppo, J.T.; van Beijsterveldt, T.C.E.M.; Boomsma, D.I. Exploring the Association between Well-Being and Psychopathology in Adolescents. *Behav. Genet.* **2013**, *43*, 177–190. [CrossRef]
41. Mojtabai, R.; Olfson, M. National Trends in Long-Term Use of Antidepressant Medications. *J. Clin. Psychiatry* **2013**, *75*, 169–177. [CrossRef]
42. Vahratian, A. Symptoms of Anxiety or Depressive Disorder and Use of Mental Health. 1 April 2021. Available online: https://www.cdc.gov/mmwr/volumes/70/wr/mm7013e2.htm (accessed on 29 September 2021).
43. Lee, J. Mental health effects of school closures during COVID-19. *Lancet Child Adolesc. Health* **2020**, *4*, 421. [CrossRef] [PubMed]
44. Loades, M.E.; Chatburn, E.; Higson-Sweeney, N.; Reynolds, S.; Shafran, R.; Brigden, A.; Linney, C.; McManus, M.N.; Borwick, C.; Crawley, E. Rapid Systematic Review: The Impact of Social Isolation and Loneliness on the Mental Health of Children and Adolescents in the Context of COVID-19. *J. Am. Acad. Child Adolesc. Psychiatry* **2020**, *59*, 1218–1239.e3. [CrossRef]
45. Racine, N.; McArthur, B.A.; Cooke, J.E.; Eirich, R.; Zhu, J.; Madigan, S. Global Prevalence of Depressive and Anxiety Symptoms in Children and Adolescents During COVID-19. *JAMA Pediatr.* **2021**, *175*, 1142. [CrossRef] [PubMed]
46. Cipriani, A.; Furukawa, T.A.; Salanti, G.; Chaimani, A.; Atkinson, L.Z.; Ogawa, Y.; Leucht, S.; Ruhe, H.G.; Turner, E.H.; Higgins, J.P.T.; et al. Comparative efficacy and acceptability of 21 antidepressant drugs for the acute treatment of adults with major depressive disorder: A systematic review and network meta-analysis. *Lancet* **2018**, *391*, 1357–1366. [CrossRef]
47. Kennedy, S.H.; Andersen, H.F.; Thase, M.E. Escitalopram in the treatment of major depressive disorder: A meta-analysis. *Curr. Med. Res. Opin.* **2008**, *25*, 161–175. [CrossRef]
48. Wade, A.G.; Crawford, G.M.; Yellowlees, A. Efficacy, safety and tolerability of escitalopram in doses up to 50 mg in Major Depressive Disorder (MDD): An open-label, pilot study. *BMC Psychiatry* **2011**, *11*, 42. [CrossRef]
49. Simon, G. *Unipolar Major Depression in Adults: Choosing Initial Treatment*; Post, T.W., Ed.; UpToDate Inc.: Waltham, MA, USA, 2023. Available online: https://www.uptodate.com/contents/unipolar-major-depression-in-adults-choosing-initial-treatment (accessed on 21 February 2023).
50. Kupka, R. *Rapid Cycling Bipolar Disorder in Adults: Treatment of Major Depression*; Post, T.W., Ed.; UpToDate Inc.: Waltham, MA, USA, 2023. Available online: https://www.uptodate.com/contents/rapid-cycling-bipolar-disorder-in-adults-treatment-of-major-depression#H92692341 (accessed on 21 February 2023).

healthcare

MDPI

Article

Health-Related Quality of Life and Healthcare Events in Patients with Monotherapy of Anti-Diabetes Medications

Tadesse Melaku Abegaz and Askal Ayalew Ali *

Economic, Social and Administrative Pharmacy (ESAP), College of Pharmacy and Pharmaceutical Sciences, Institute of Public Heath, Florida A&M University, Tallahassee, FL 32307, USA
* Correspondence: askal.ali@famu.edu

Abstract: This study aimed to examine the difference in health-related quality of life (HRQOL) and diabetes-related healthcare events (HCEs) among adults with diabetes who were on metformin, sulfonylurea, insulin, or thiazolidinedione (TZD) monotherapy. The data were sourced from the Medical Expenditure Panel Survey (MEPS). Diabetes patients ≥18 years old who had a complete record of physical component score and mental component scores in round 2 and round 4 of the survey were included. The primary outcome was HRQOL of diabetes patients as measured by the Medical Outcome Study short-form (SF-12v2^{TM}). Multinomial logistic regression and negative binomial regression were conducted to determine associated factors of HRQOL and HCE, respectively. Overall, 5387 patients were included for analysis. Nearly 60% of patients had unchanged HRQOL after the follow-up, whereas almost 15% to 20% of patients showed improvement in HRQOL. The relative risk of declined mental HRQOL was 1.5 times higher relative to unchanged mental HRQOL in patients who were on sulfonylurea 1.55 [1.1–2.17, p = 0.01] than metformin users. The rate of HCE decreased by a factor of 0.79, [95% CI: 0.63–0.99] in patients with no history of hypertension. Patients on sulfonylurea 1.53 [1.20–1.95, <0.01], insulin 2.00 [1.55–2.70, <0.01], and TZD 1.78 [1.23–2.58, <0.01] had increased risk of HCE compared to patients who were on metformin. In general, antidiabetic medications modestly improved HRQOL in patients with diabetes during the follow-up period. Metformin had a lower rate of HCE as compared to other medications. The selection of anti-diabetes medications should focus on HRQOL in addition to controlling glucose level.

Keywords: anti-diabetes medications; comparative effectiveness; diabetes; quality of life

Citation: Abegaz, T.M.; Ali, A.A. Health-Related Quality of Life and Healthcare Events in Patients with Monotherapy of Anti-Diabetes Medications. *Healthcare* **2023**, *11*, 541. https://doi.org/10.3390/healthcare11040541

Academic Editor: Ioannis Ilias

Received: 31 December 2022
Revised: 6 February 2023
Accepted: 9 February 2023
Published: 12 February 2023

1. Introduction

It is predicted that the number of patients suffering from diabetes mellitus (DM) will increase to 366 million in 2030 globally [1]. In the United States (US), DM affects more than 10% of the population [2]. DM causes multiple complications, including cardiovascular, renal, eye, and extremities. It has been revealed that DM and its complications are negatively associated with the health-related quality of life (HRQOL) of patients [3].

Pharmacotherapeutic interventions play a pivotal role in controlling high glucose, preventing diabetes-related complications, improving survival, and improving HRQOL of patients with diabetes [4,5]. Metformin, sulfonylurea, insulin, and thiazolidinediones (TZD) are the commonly used anti-diabetes medications. The American Diabetes Association (ADA) recommends these medications as the first-line therapy owing to their affordability and proved safety [6]. Previous studies in the US also reported that the use of metformin and insulin analogues increased from 1999 to 2018, derived from an ongoing safety and effectiveness study on these agents [7,8]. Despite extensive research on the glycemic effects of these first-line medications, their impact on HRQOL has yet to be explored in a real-world scenario. In addition to the aforementioned glucose-lowering agents, several hypoglycemic agents have been approved for the management of diabetes most recently. Even though the introduction of newer glucose-lowering agents such as GLP-1 agonists and SGLT2 inhibitors improves the management of DM, they are usually prescribed as a second-line therapy in the case of uncontrolled diabetes. In addition, the high cost of these medications limits their utilization for patients mainly with cardiorenal complications [9].

Few clinical trials studies have integrated patient-reported outcomes measures to evaluate the effectiveness of different pharmacotherapeutic interventions on HRQOL [10–13]. However, the generalizability of these clinical trials is limited. Meraya et al. (2020) reported poor HRQOL in patients with diabetes complications using the Medical Expenditure Panel Survey (MEPS) data [14]. A study conducted by Campbell et al. (2017) revealed that HRQOL of patients with diabetes declined as the medical expenditure of patients with diabetes increased [15]. However, these studies did not compare the effect of treatments on HRQOL and the difference in effectiveness across various anti-diabetes medications. In addition, there are limited data on diabetes-related healthcare events (HCEs), including emergency, inpatient, and outpatient visits in patients who use selected anti-diabetes medications.

The aim of this study was twofold: (1) to explore the difference in HRQOL in patients who were on monotherapy of the common anti-diabetes treatments; (2) to investigate healthcare events associated with diabetes across diabetes treatments. Investigation of the HRQOL of interventions would improve decision making during prescription by providing evidence on the comparative effectiveness of diabetes treatments.

2. Materials and Methods

2.1. Study Design and Population

A longitudinal study was conducted on non-institutionalized US civilian diabetes patients using the Medical Expenditure Panel Survey (MEPS), a nationally representative survey from 2000–2019 [16]. MEPS collects data from each participant in five consecutive rounds. Information on HRQOL is only collected in rounds 2 and 4. In each round, information on prescribed medicines is recorded including name, price, dose, and prescription dates.

Our study population included all diabetes patients above the age of 18 who participated in the MEPS survey in rounds 2 and 4, which were approximately 1 year apart. Participants who started their medication prior to round 2 were eligible to participate in the study, allowing for the measurement of changes in HRQOL between rounds 2 and 4. All eligible patients were also required to have a complete record of HRQOL. In addition, diabetes patients who received only monotherapy of metformin, sulfonylurea, insulin, or TZD were included in the study. Our exclusion criteria were patients who purchased their medication between rounds 3 and round 5, patients on combination glucose-lowering agents, patients with an incomplete record of HRQOL, and patients who changed therapy between the two rounds.

2.2. Primary Outcomes and Study Variables

The primary outcome of this study was HRQOL of diabetes patients who were on common antidiabetic medicines. The secondary outcome constituted HCEs, which included home health events, outpatient events, inpatient events, emergency room events, and hospitalizations associated with diabetes. The "home health events" variable in MEPS encompasses data on the use of in-home health services, including home health visits, hospice care, and other medical treatments provided in a person's residence. This variable provides insights into the type, frequency, and cost of home health services received by individuals, enabling the analysis of trends and patterns in the utilization and spending of home health services. Inpatient events and hospitalizations include diabetes-related complications such as diabetic ketoacidosis, myocardial infarctions, stroke, foot, or urinary tract infections. All other events related to diabetes but not requiring admission to the hospital were categorized under outpatient visit such as kidney, cholesterol, eye, and hemoglobin A1C exams. The reason for all events was the diabetic condition.

The independent variables were sociodemographic characteristics of patients including sex, age, race, ethnicity, marital status, employment status, and education. Comorbidity conditions such as coronary heart disease, asthma, hypertension, angina, stroke, myocardial infarction, emphysema, arthritis, cancer, and dyslipidemia were included as additional explanatory variables.

2.3. Data Source and Data Collection

We used data from Medical Expenditure Panel Survey Household Component (MEPS-HC). The household component of MEPS consists of data collected from each household member on demographic characteristics, medical conditions, health status, events, prescription medicines, and medical expenses. The four classes of glucose-lowering agents were retrieved from the prescription medication file, which provides information about the therapeutic classes of medicines in connection with the Multum Lexicon database. The diagnosis of DM and other conditions was identified from the medical condition file.

The HRQOL was measured using the Medical Outcome Study 12 Item Short-Form (SF-12v2^{TM}), a standardized generic questionnaire of medical outcome study which contains 12 items. Since 2000, SF-12v2^{TM} has been administered to adults above 18 years old. The SF-12v2 was validated using MEPS for measuring HLQOL in diabetic patients in the US (Cronbach α: PCS = 0.85; MCS = 0.83) [17]. It was also validated to measure HRQOL by Ware et al. in the general population [18]. The eight domains of SF-12v2^{TM} are summarized into two components: the physical component score (PCS) and the mental component score (MCS). The MCS and PCS are scored out of 100. Higher scores are associated with better physical and mental health. An average score of both MCS and PCS is 50 points for the general US population [18]. For the purpose of this study, classification of the HRQOL status was carried out using the minimum clinically important difference (MCID) method, which is described below.

2.4. Minimum Clinically Important Difference in HRQOL

We computed the MCID to determine whether the change in HRQOL between round 2 (before treatment) and round 4 (after treatment) was clinically meaningful [19]. MCID can be computed using different approaches. The distribution-based approach is the common method that estimates MCID using different measures. The half standard deviation (half-SD) is utilized as a common distribution-based method. According to previous studies, a value of half-SD approximates the threshold of discrimination for clinically meaningful changes in HRQOL for chronic diseases [20,21]. The half-SD is estimated by calculating the SD of the change in MCS and PCS scores between the two rounds. Then, HRQOL is categorized into improved, unchanged, and declined on the basis of the values of the half-SD.

2.5. Data Analyses

Data were cleaned and analyzed using Stata Version 15 [22]. All analyses were conducted using survey procedures. The present study considers the sampling weights (longitudinal weights), clustering, and stratification design to determine HRQOL and diabetes-related events. Descriptive statistics were performed on the patient's demographic and clinical characteristics, while multinomial logistic regression was conducted to determine association between the different classes of medications and HRQOL. The categorical forms of the mental and physical components of HRQOL were our dependent variables. Negative binomial regression was conducted to assess factors associated with HCE. HCE was a count variable with unequal mean and variance. The negative binomial model was the best fit model for such data. A p-value < 0.05 was set a priori with a 95% confidence interval to test the level of significance.

3. Results

3.1. Characteristics of Diabetes Patients

Overall, 5387 individuals met the inclusion criteria (weighted estimate: 103,169,500). Overall, 50% of participants were males (49.33%). The mean age of participants was 60.65 (SD: 20.78). More than three-fourths of the participants were non-Hispanic whites (73.53%). The majority were married (58.25%). Almost 19% of patients had health insurance. About 40% of them were employed. Approximately 11% had stroke, 12% had asthma, and one-half of the participants (49.92%) had arthritis. More than 70% of the population had dyslipidemia (73.18%). Three-fourths (75.15%) of the subjects had high blood pressure. There was a significant difference among participants in the four medication groups in terms of sex, race, marital status, ethnicity, age as a categorical variable, stroke, angina, high cholesterol, arthritis, and diabetes-related eye complications ($p < 0.01$), whereas no significant differences were reported in other characteristics, including education, health insurance, coronary heart disease, high blood pressure, emphysema, and asthma (Table 1).

Table 1. Characteristics of the study participants, Wt (%).

Variables	Metformin	Sulfonylurea	Insulin	TZD	Total	*p*-Value
Sex						
Male	13.65	16.51	10.57	8.6	49.33	0.02
Female	16.24	15.11	10.55	8.76	50.67	
Age (mean ± SD)	58.68 (32.85)	63.3 (31)	58.44 (45.45)	61.87 (34.6)	60.65 (20.78)	0.5144
18–39	2.42	1.4	2.78	0.56	7.16	
40–49	4.91	3.65	2.94	2.03	13.52	
50–59	7.97	6.81	4.31	4.58	23.67	<0.01
60–69	7.91	8.81	5.27	5.59	27.57	
70+	36.69	10.95	5.83	4.61	28.07	
Race						
White	21.99	22.83	14.31	14.39	73.53	
Black	4.46	4.66	4.37	2.45	15.93	<0.01
American Indian	0.35	0.53	0.27	0.23	1.38	
Asian	1.36	1.69	0.64	0.63	4.33	
Native Hawaiian/Pacific Islander	0.83	1.42	0.71	0.3	3.25	
Others	0.49	0.43	0.3	0.36	1.58	
Ethnicity						
Hispanic	4.41	5.05	2.57	2.39	14.42	
NH Black	8.99	8.49	7.19	3.11	27.79	<0.01
NH Asian	2.7	3.44	1.91	0.96	9	
NH white	13.5	14.32	9.29	10.85	47.95	
NH other	0.29	0.32	0.17	0.05	0.84	
Marital status						
Married	16.52	18.6	11.65	11.48	58.25	0.04
Widowed	4.02	5.56	3.15	3.04	15.74	
Divorced	3.91	4.18	2.82	2.62	13.53	
Separated	0.6	0.7	0.64	0.53	2.48	
Never married	2.76	2.31	2.73	2.19	2.19	
Education						
No degree	6.75	7.67	4.56	3.66	22.64	0.707
High school diploma	15.09	16.82	11.81	8.65	52.37	
Bachelor's degree and above	7.57	7.26	5.45	4.71	24.99	
Health insurance status (Yes)	27.77	28.71	17.89	14.21	88.57	0.496
Comorbidity						
Coronary heart disease	3.69	5.65	5.18	3.15	0.68	0.68
Asthma	4.05	3.82	3.15	1.5	12.52	0.612
Hypertension	21.7	24.68	15.6	13.17	75.15	0.194
Angina	2.13	2.55	1.89	9.35	15.92	<0.01
Myocardial infarction	3.14	4.99	3.89	2.16	14.17	<0.01
Stroke	2.5	3.65	3.3	1.69	11.14	<0.01
Emphysema	1.34	1.76	0.9	0.61	4.61	0.417
Arthritis	14.41	15.81	10.51	9.19	49.92	0.106
Dyslipidaemia	21.87	23.29	15.02	13	73.18	<0.01
Cancer	5.00	6.24	5.05	2.77	19.06	0.042
Employment (yes)	15.31	11.53	8.27	7.71	42.83	<0.01

Wt: weighted, TZD: thiazolidinedione, NH: non-Hispanic, SD: standard deviation.

3.2. Health-Related Quality of Life of Diabetes Patients

More than 60% of patients had unchanged status in mental-HRQOL (62.91%) and physical-HRQOL (67.02%) components, whereas almost 15% to 20% of patients showed an improvement in HRQOL for all monotherapy users as compared to the baseline (Table 2). The maximum improvement in HRQOL among individual antidiabetic medications did not exceed 5% between the two periods, and the HRQOL improvement was comparable across medications. In the metformin group, 4.76% and 4.1% of individuals had improved in MCS and PCS components, respectively. The improvement in HRQOL in the insulin group ranged from 4.7% on MCS and 4.78% on PCS. In the sulfonylurea group, the improvement in HRQOL was between 4.57% and 5.59% (Table 2).

Table 2. Health-related quality of life of diabetes patients.

Treatments	MCS Wt (%)			PCS Wt (%)		
	Improved	Unchanged	Declined	Improved	Unchanged	Declined
Metformin	4.76	19.86	5.27	4.1	20.53	5.26
Sulfonylureas	5.59	19.46	6.58	4.57	20.8	6.25
Insulin	3.7	12.51	4.47	3.78	13.51	3.84
TZD	2.82	11.09	3.46	2.22	12.18	2.94
Total	20.23	62.91	16.86	14.7	67.02	18.28

MCS: mental component score, PCS: physical component score, TZD: thiazolidinedione, Wt: weighted.

The overall trend of HRQOL increased slightly in the MCS component across different panels with an overall mean ± SD of 45.55 ± 15.77 (interquartile range = 38.51–57.16). A sharp decline in MCS was observed in panel 19 (mean MCS = 40.652) (Table 2). The trend of the PCS score remained stable across different panels (mean ± SD = 37.679 ± 15.19, interquartile range = 27.751–50.22) (Figures 1 and 2).

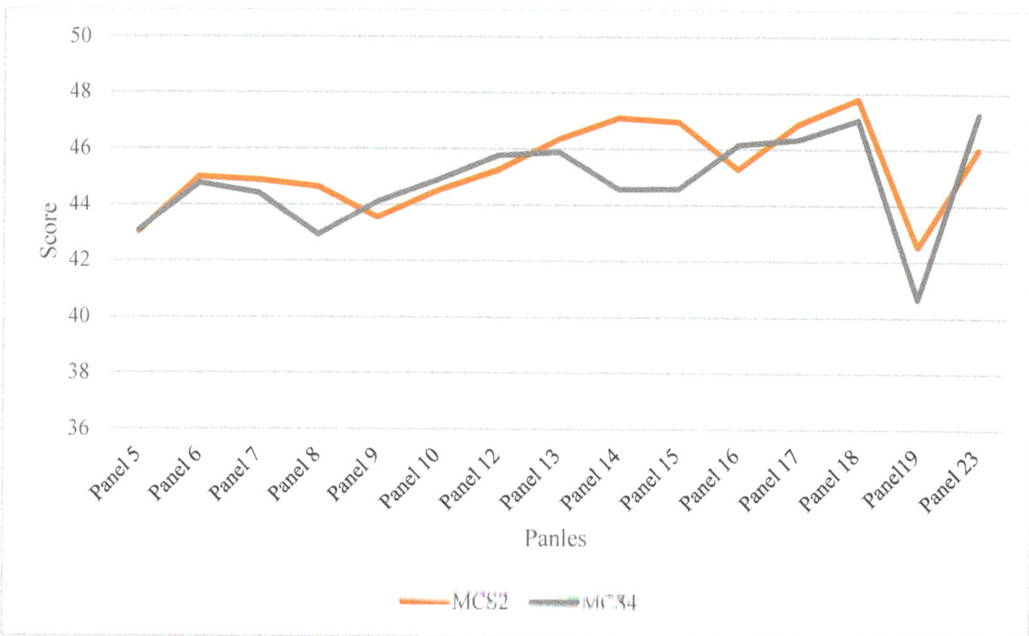

Figure 1. The trend of mental component score (MCS) domain: Panels 11, 20, 21, and 22 are not shown in the graph due to an incomplete record of HRQOL. MCS2: mental component score in round 2, MCS4: mental component score in round 4.

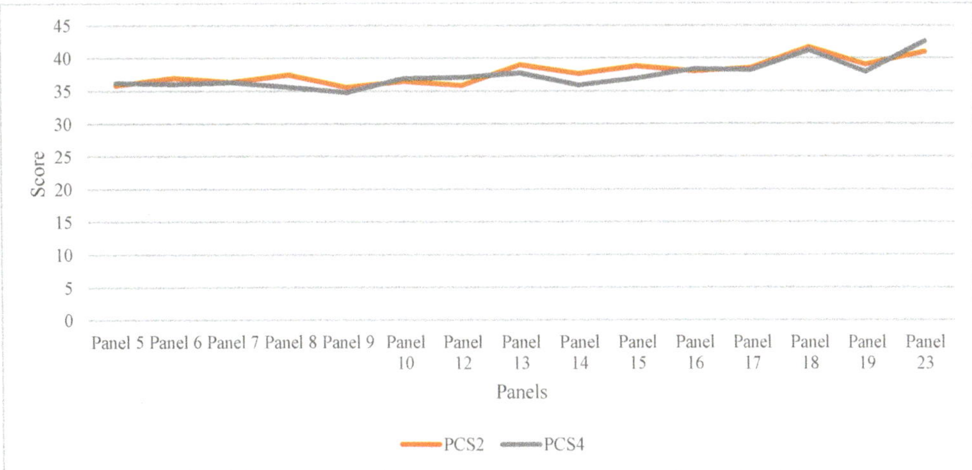

Figure 2. The trend of physical component score (PCS) domain, panels 5–23. Panels 11, 20, 21, and 22 are not shown in the graph due to an incomplete record of HRQOL. PCS2: physical component score in round 2, PCS4: physical component score in round 4.

3.3. Factors Associated with Health-Related Quality of Life of Diabetes Patients

To determine factors associated with HROQL, we ran a multinomial logistic regression. It was found that, among many factors, age, race, and antidiabetic medications were found to be associated with HRQOL. The relative risk for improved mental HRQOL status relative to unchanged status increased by 50% in patients aged 40 to 49 and 60 to 69 years old (0.53 [95 CI% 0.27–0.92, $p = 0.02$] and 0.50 [95 CI% 0.32–0.98, $p = 0.02$], respectively), as compared with patients aged between 18 and 39. Relative to Hispanics, the relative risk of improved mental HRQOL relative to unchanged mental HRQOL was 48% lower for Blacks 0.52 [0.34–0.79, <0.01] and 55% lower for NH whites 0.45 [0.28–0.73, <0.01]. The relative risk of declined mental HRQOL as compared to unchanged mental HRQOL increased by 1.45 in patients with a history of unemployment 1.45 [1.02–2.04, 0.03] as compared with employed individuals. The relative risk of declined mental HRQOL was 1.5 times higher relative to unchanged mental HRQOL in patients who were on sulfonylurea than metformin users 1.55 [1.1–2.17, $p = 0.01$]. In comparison to Hispanics, non-Hispanic whites had 40% less risk of improved physical HRQOL 0.60 [0.41–0.90, $p = 0.01$] relative to unchanged physical HRQOL. In contrast to the Hispanic population, Black patients had about 37% lower risk of improved physical HRQOL relative to unchanged physical HRQOL (0.63 [0.41–0.96, $p = 0.03$]). Patients with the age range of 50–59 had almost 45% lower risk of improved physical HRQOL relative to unchanged physical HRQOL (0.55 [0.31–0.96, $p = 0.04$]; Tables 3 and 4).

Table 3. Factors affecting mental HRQOL of diabetes patients.

Variables	**Declined**		**Improved**	
	RRR 95% CI	***p*-Value**	**RRR 95% CI**	***p*-Value**
Sex (Ref: male)				
Female	1.13 [0.8430–1.53]	0.4	1.22 [0.88–1.69]	0.22
Age (Ref: 18–39)				
40–49	0.62 [0.33–1.18]	0.14	0.53 [0.27–0.92]	0.02
50–59	0.92 [0.51–1.65]	0.78	0.74 [0.44–1.24]	0.25
60–69	0.77 [0.42–1.42]	0.4	0.50 [0.32–0.98]	0.02
70+	0.81 [0.45–1.44]	0.47	0.76 [0.43–1.35]	0.35
Race (Ref: Hispanic)				
NH Black	0.82 [0.56–1.2]	0.31	0.52 [0.34–0.79]	<0.01
NH Asian	0.95 [0.61–1.49]	0.82	0.99 [0.64–1.52]	0.96
NH white	0.87 [0.55–1.38]	0.56	0.45 [0.28–0.73]	<0.01
NH others	1.16 [0.46–2.92]	0.46	1.17 [0.38–3.59]	0.78

Table 3. *Cont.*

Variables	Declined		Improved	
	RRR 95% CI	***p*-Value**	**RRR 95% CI**	***p*-Value**
Insurance (Ref: yes)				
No	1.31 [0.83–2.05]	0.24	1.1 [0.65–1.8]	0.76
Employment (Ref: yes)				
No	1.45 [1.02–2.04]	0.03	1.08 [0.77–1.5]	0.8
Coronary artery disease (Ref: yes)				
No	1.032 [0.63–1.69]	0.89	0.86 [0.54–1.36]	0.51
Asthma (Ref: yes)				
No	0.81 [0.54–1.19]	0.28	1.22 [0.77–1.92]	0.39
Hypertension (Ref: yes)				
No	0.88 [0.61–1.27]	0.5	0.94 [0.63–1.4]	0.78
Angina (Ref: yes)				
No	0.85 [0.48–1.48]	0.56	0.93 [0.54–1.58]	0.78
Myocardial infarction (Ref: yes)				
No	0.82 [0.45–1.47]	0.51	1.13 [0.66–1.93]	0.64
Emphysema (Ref: yes)				
No	0.61 [0.31–1.18]	0.14	0.64 [0.29–1.43]	0.27
Dyslipidaemia (Ref: yes)				
No	1.32 [0.89–1.97]	0.16	0.85 [0.57–1.25]	0.41
Cancer (Ref: yes)				
No	0.76 [0.54–1.05]	0.1	1.14 [0.76–1.71]	0.51
Arthritis (Ref: yes)				
No	0.83 [0.58–1.17]	0.29	0.82 [0.56–1.19]	0.3
Healthcare events (Ref: 0)				
One events	0.84 [0.51–1.39]	0.4	0.76 [0.49–1.18]	0.22
2–3 events	0.8 [0.52–1.23]	0.32	1.11 [0.74–1.66]	0.60
4–5 events	0.79 [0.43–1.46]	0.46	1.08 [0.6–1.96]	0.77
≥6 events	0.89 [0.55–1.42]	0.62	0.91 [0.55–1.5]	0.72
Anti-diabetes (Ref: metformin)				
Sulfonylureas	1.55 [1.1–2.17]	0.01	1.11 [0.72–1.73]	0.62
Insulin	1.39 [0.88–2.22]	0.15	1.09 [0.70–1.68]	0.70
TZD	1.69 [1–2.89]	0.05	0.94 [0.55–1.6]	0.55

NH: Non-Hispanic, RRR: relative risk ratio, TZD: thiazolidinedione.

Table 4. Factors affecting physical HRQOL of diabetes patients.

Variables	Declined		Improved	
	RRR 95% CI	***p*-Value**	**RRR 95% CI**	***p*-Value**
Sex (Ref: male)				
Female	0.93 [0.69–1.28]	0.69	1.35 [0.9–1.9]	0.06
Age (Ref: 18–39)				
40–49	0.73 [0.38–1.4]	0.35	0.80 [0.42–1.5]	0.50
50–59	0.81 [0.47–1.4]	0.44	0.55 [0.31–0.96]	0.04
60–69	0.72 [0.42–1.2]	0.22	0.84 [0.48–1.47]	0.55
70+	1.06 [0.38–1.4]	0.9	0.70 [0.39–1.27]	0.25
Race (Ref: Hispanic)				
NH Black	1.04 [0.71–1.54]	0.82	0.63 [0.41–0.96]	0.03
NH Asian	0.81 [0.53–1.3]	0.36	0.98 [0.64–1.48]	0.9
NH white	0.78 [0.51–1.19]	0.25	0.60 [0.41–0.90]	0.01
NH others	1.16 [0.39–2.8]	0.46	0.93 [0.41–2.08]	0.85
Insurance (Ref: yes)				
No	1.19 [0.69–2.06]	0.52	1.39 [0.93–2.11]	0.11
Employment (Ref: yes)				
No	1.42 [0.94–2.15]	0.09	1.02 [0.69–1.3]	0.64
Coronary artery disease (Ref: yes)				
No	0.7 [0.46–1.1]	0.11	1.1 [0.70–1.75]	0.7
Asthma (Ref: yes)				
No	1.1 [0.74–1.58]	0.69	0.86 [0.52–1.82]	0.55
Angina (Ref: yes)				
No	1.1 [0.64–1.9]	0.72	0.65 [0.40–1.03]	0.07
Myocardial infarction (Ref: yes)				
No	0.83 [0.50–1.38]	0.48	0.74 [0.42–1.3]	0.30
Emphysema (Ref: yes)				
No	0.67 [0.36–1.22]	0.19	0.05 [0.16–1.56]	[illegible]
Dyslipidaemia (Ref: yes)				
No	0.87 [0.57–1.33]	0.49	1 [0.66–1.25]	0.98
Cancer (Ref: yes)				
No	1.08 [0.54–1.05]	0.8	0.9 [0.57–1.1]	0.63
Healthcare events (Ref: 0)				
One events	0.7 [0.47–1.05]	0.09	0.81 [0.50–1.13]	0.39
2–3 events	0.65 [0.42–1]	0.05	0.81 [0.52–1.4]	0.36
4–5 events	0.62 [0.35–1.08]	0.09	0.90 [0.48–1.7]	0.72
≥6 events	0.73 [0.43–1.24]	0.24	0.82 [0.49–1.37]	0.44
Anti-diabetes (Ref: metformin)				
Sulfonylureas	1.31 [0.88–1.94]	0.17	0.89 [0.62–1.28]	0.53
Insulin	0.98 [0.59–1.6]	0.92	0.96 [0.65–1.41]	0.84
TZD	1.04 [0.62–1.74]	0.89	0.78 [0.43–1.42]	0.43

RRR: relative risk ratio, TZD: thiazolidinedione.

3.4. Healthcare-Associated Events in Diabetes Patients

One-quarter of patients had no healthcare-associated events (23.46%). About one-fifth (18.85%) of patients had greater than six events. Around 18.2% of patients had at least one HCE. There was a significant difference among participants who received different anti-diabetes treatments in terms of the number of HCEs associated with diabetes, including emergency visits, home health visits, inpatient events, and office-based events ($p < 0.01$). No significant difference was observed between different treatment groups regarding hospital stay and outpatient events (Table 5).

Table 5. The mean number of healthcare-associated events in diabetes patients across different treatments.

Type of Events	Metformin	Sulfonylurea	Insulin	TZD	Total	p-Value
Emergency events	0.03	0.03	0.09	0.02	0.17	<0.01
Home health events	0.11	0.15	0.27	0.16	0.69	<0.01
Hospital stays	0	0.03	0	0.18	0.21	0.18
Inpatient events	0.01	0.02	0.08	0.01	0.12	<0.01
Office-based events	2.24	2.86	3.55	3.51	12.16	<0.01
Outpatient events	0.13	0.16	0.23	0.27	0.79	0.08
Number of HCEs						
No event	8.89	7.5	4.18	2.88	23.46	
One events	6.24	5.72	3.49	2.76	18.2	
2–3 events	7.59	7.99	5.06	4.59	25.23	<0.01
4–5 events	3.44	4.86	2.86	3.12	14.26	
≥6 events	3.73	5.55	5.54	4.03	18.85	

HCEs: healthcare events, TZD: thiazolidinedione.

3.5. Determinants of Healthcare Events Associated with Diabetes

According to the result of the negative binomial regression model, the most significant determinant factors associated with the occurrence of HCEs are shown in Table 6. Compared with married individuals, being widowed increased the risk of HCEs by a factor of 1.46 [1.02–2.1, $p < 0.01$]. Relative to employed individuals, patients without employment had 1.44 times greater rate for HCE [1.16–1.79, $p = 0.01$]. The rate of HCEs decreased by a factor of 0.79 in patients without a history of hypertension compared hypertensive patients [0.63–0.99, $p = 0.04$]. Patients on sulfonylurea (1.53 [1.20–1.95, <0.01]), insulin (2.00 [1.55–2.70, <0.01]), and TZD (1.78 [1.23–2.58, <0.01]) had increased risk of HCEs compared to patients who were on metformin (Table 6).

Table 6. Determinants of healthcare events associated with diabetes: negative binomial regression model.

Factors	IRR 95%CI	p-Value
Sex (Ref: male)		
Female	0.98 [0.81–1.2]	0.88
Age (Ref: 18–39)		
40–49	1.32 [0.89–1.94]	0.16
50–59	1.13 [0.79–1.61]	0.5
60–69	0.96 [0.66–1.34]	0.82
+70	0.78 [0.55–1.13]	0.19
Race (Ref: Hispanic)		
NH Black	0.94 [0.77–1.14]	0.53
NH Asian	0.83 [0.62–1.1]	0.5
NH white	1.12 [0.75–1.66]	0.57
NH others	0.74 [0.44–1.2]	0.27
Marital status (Ref: married)		
Widowed	1.46 [1.02–2.1]	0.04
Divorced	1.14 [0.85–1.53]	0.37
Separated	0.95 [0.6–1.48]	0.81
Never married	0.99 [0.75–1.32]	0.94

Table 6. *Cont.*

Factors	IRR 95%CI	*p*-Value
Insurance (Ref: yes)		
No	1.33 [0.96–1.85]	0.08
Employment (Ref: yes)		
No	1.44 [1.16–1.79]	0.01
Coronary artery disease (Ref: yes)		
No	1.03 [0.72–1.47]	0.88
Asthma		
No	1.29 [0.94–1.79]	0.11
Hypertension (Ref: yes)		
No	0.79 [0.63–0.99]	0.04
Angina (Ref: yes)		
No	0.92 [0.61–1.38]	0.68
Stroke (Ref: yes)		
No	1.12 [0.87–1.44]	0.4
Dyslipidaemia (Ref: yes)		
No	1.19 [0.91–1.55]	0.19
Cancer (Ref: yes)		
No	1.2 [0.94–1.54]	0.15
Arthritis (Ref: yes)		
No	0.80 [0.67–0.96]	0.02
Anti-diabetes (Ref: metformin)		
Sulfonylureas	1.53 [1.20–1.95]	<0.01
Insulin	2.00 [1.55–2.70]	<0.01
TZD	1.78 [1.23–2.58]	<0.01

IRR: incidence rate ratio, NH: non-Hispanic, TZD: thiazolidinedione.

4. Discussion

Most studies have focused on the evaluation of intermediate clinical endpoints of diabetes (i.e., glycemic control) following anti-diabetes treatments. Recently, a few comparative effectiveness studies integrated patient reported outcomes measures along with randomized control trial studies to measure HRQOL [10–13]. However, a real-world evaluation of HRQOL of diabetes patients on different treatment modalities has not been sufficiently explored [23]. This study aimed to evaluate the HRQOL and HCE of patients with diabetes who were taking selected anti-diabetes treatments.

According to our findings, about 15–20% of patients showed an improvement in HRQOL from the baseline HRQOL level. More than 20% of the population had unchanged HRQOL at the end of the follow-up. The trend in HRQOL did not show a significant change across different panels in physical HERQOL, but a sharp decline was observed in mental HRQOL from panels 18 to 19 before increasing afterward. Several factors were associated with poor HRQOL, including history of unemployment, type of anti-diabetes, Black and white races, and age ranges of 40–49 and 60–69. More than 20% of diabetes individuals experienced at least one HCE associated with diabetes. Multiple factors influenced the occurrence of HCEs in diabetes patients such as marital status, employment status, and anti-diabetes medications.

Our study indicated that the use of anti diabetes medications modestly improved HRQOL in diabetes patients. This could be through achieving adequate glycemic control [24,25]. The effectiveness of these medications to improve HRQOL could also be attributed to preventing diabetes-related complications [26,27]. For instance, TZDs were reported to confer cardioprotective effect. According to recent studies, TZDs such as pioglitazone significantly improve endothelial and adipose tissue dysfunction and reduce the composite of nonfatal myocardial infarction and stroke in patients with type 2 diabetes, which might contribute to HRQOL improvement [28,29]. However, there is controversy about the role of TZD on CVD outcomes as they were once labeled as a black-box warning for worsening of heart failure in in diabetes patients [30]. On the other hand, evidence on the effects of sulfonylureas on the heart is still not conclusive and remains an ongoing debate [31]. The modest improvement in HRQOL associated with the use of these glucose-lowering agents might also be ascribed to the use of a single blood glucose-lowering agent. Rizza et al. (2021) noted that using a single dose of anti-diabetes medication resulted in a greater likelihood of improving health and quality of life as compared to combination therapies [32]. Additional pharmacotherapeutic properties of individual anti-diabetes medications could also contribute to their impact on HRQOL. For example, metformin decreases obesity, which might affect physical health. However, some safety profiles, such as undesired weight gain due to insulin and sulfonylurea might attenuate their benefit on HRQOL [33,34]. Weight gain has a negative psychological impact and compromises physical strength, which might expose one to frailty [35]. As noted in the multinomial regression report, a relatively higher rate of decline in HRQOL associated with sulfonylureas and TZD as compared to metformin could be attributed to safety differences between treatments [36]. However, controlled studies with an adequate follow-up period are required to capture the difference in HRQOL between these agents.

The current study explored the magnitude of improvement in HRQOL as influenced by race and ethnicity. Black Americans and NH whites had a higher rate of decline in HRQOL. The disparity in HRQOL might be due to the variation in response to anti-diabetes medications between different racial/ethnic groups and the difference in socioeconomic status [37]. Even though patients had equal probability of taking anti-diabetes medications, the difference in economic status could affect access to psychological services, especially for African-Americans [38]. Despite the socioeconomic disadvantages surrounding the Hispanic population, Hispanics in the United States tend to have significantly better health outcomes than the average population, which was also observed in our study [39]. The present study also reported variation in the HRQOL between different age groups. It was found that middle-aged to older individuals tended to have lower HRQOL than young patients [40]. As age increased, the number of comorbidities and healthcare events become more pronounced, resulting in decreased HRQOL [41]. On the other hand, some studies reported that HRQOL was better in older patients, which might be related to the high amount of healthcare received by the older population [38–42].

In the present study, one in five individuals had at least one HCE associated with diabetes. As with many chronic conditions, diabetes is known to cause multiple inpatient and outpatient events [43]. A number of studies reported that patients with diabetes had a 2–6 times higher rate of admission than patients without diabetes [44,45]. In 2015, it was estimated that 92 in 1000 diabetes patients would visit an emergency room in the US [46]. HCEs related to diabetes can occur at the onset of the disease in the form of diabetic ketoacidosis or micro- and macrovascular complications. The frequent precipitation of hyperglycemia and the progression of the disease add a tally to several admissions [47]. The occurrence of these events might vary according to the type of pharmacologic management. In our study, it was stated that the use of sulfonylureas, insulin, and TZD was likely to increase the rate of HCEs as compared to metformin. The high rate of HCEs in these medications could be inadequate glucose control when given as monotherapy [48]. Poor insulin administration might also exacerbate hyperglycemia and emergency visits [44]. Roumie et al. (2012) reported that the use of sulfonylureas for the treatment of diabetes was associated with an increased hazard of diabetes-related events (18.2 per 1000 person-years) compared to metformin users (10.4 per 1000 person-years) [49]. Lipscombe et al. (2007) reported that treatment with TZD monotherapy was associated with a significantly increased risk of congestive heart failure, acute myocardial infarction, and death compared with other oral hypoglycemic therapies that led to emergency room visits [50]. Thus, HCEs associated with diabetes could be mitigated with the appropriate selection of anti-diabetes medications.

In general, the present study provided important information on HRQOL and HCEs in patients with diabetes who were on different anti-diabetes medications. The representativeness of the sample could allow generalizability of the findings. However, the retrospective design of the study did not enable to control all confounders of HRQOL. In addition, the duration of therapy between the two timepoints may not have been able to capture significant differences in HRQOL between the two rounds. The HRQOL assessment tool is not specific to diabetes, which could also have affected our estimation of HRQOL in these special population. The study was also affected by bias from self-reported HRQOL. Our study did not incorporate the impact of nonpharmacological interventions that might influence HRQOL. The current study did not evaluate the difference in HRQOL of other anti-diabetes medications such as sodium glucose transporter inhibiters and incretin mimetics that are usually combined with one or more of selected anti-diabetes medications. The findings of the study should be interpreted in light of these limitations.

5. Conclusions and Recommendations

In conclusion, antidiabetic medications modestly improved HRQOL in patients with diabetes during the follow-up period. The overall improvement in HRQOL was approximately 20%. Patients with sulfonylurea had a higher decline in HRQOL. Patients on metformin had a lower rate of HCEs as compared to other medications. There was a difference in HRQOL in terms of race and age. The selection of anti-diabetes medication should focus on HRQOL in addition to intermediate outcomes (i.e., glucose level). Special attention is required for patients with various age groups and ethnic origins to improve HRQOL in patients with diabetes. Policymakers should ensure the availability of glucose-lowering agents that demonstrate high yield of HRQOL at affordable price. The enrolment of diabetes patients to different health plans such as traditional Medicare versus Medicare advantage could cause variation in the uptake of anti-diabetes medications [51]. Efforts should be sought to eliminate disparity in receiving these glucose-lowering agents across diabetes patients who are enrolled in different health plans. Engagement of patients' view during drug selection could also help to initiate appropriate anti-diabetes medication with better HRQOL. Future research can be directed to comparing the HRQOL of patients taking combination therapies with respect to other new therapeutic alternatives such as GLP-1 agonists and SGLT2 inhibitors.

Author Contributions: Conceptualization, T.M.A. and A.A.A.; methodology, T.M.A. and A.A.A.; software, T.M.A.; validation, T.M.A. and A.A.A.; formal analysis, T.M.A.; investigation; T.M.A. and A.A.A.; resources, T.M.A. and A.A.A.; data curation, T.M.A.; writing—original draft preparation, T.M.A.; writing—review and editing, T.M.A. and A.A.A.; visualization, T.M.A.; supervision, A.A.A.; project administration, T.M.A. and A.A.A. All authors have read and agreed to the published version of the manuscript.

Funding: This research received no external funding.

Institutional Review Board Statement: The study was deemed exempt by the Florida A&M University IRB committee with reference number 095-22.

Informed Consent Statement: Informed consent was not applicable since the present study accessed data from MEPS which is a secondary data source.

Data Availability Statement: Not applicable.

Acknowledgments: The authors would like to acknowledge Florida A&M University for overall support. This study was supported by departmental funding-Title III program in the FAMU College of Pharmacy and Pharmaceutical Sciences, Institute of Public Health (CoPPS, IPH). We would like to extend our gratitude to patients who participated in MEPS. All individuals who are included in this section have consented to the acknowledgement.

Conflicts of Interest: The authors declare no conflict of interest.

References

1. Wild, S.; Roglic, G.; Green, A.; Sicree, R.; King, H. Global prevalence of diabetes: Estimates for the year 2000 and projections for 2030. *Diabetes Care* **2004**, *27*, 1047–1053. [CrossRef]
2. Engelgau, M.M.; Geiss, L.S.; Saaddine, J.B.; Boyle, J.P.; Benjamin, S.M.; Gregg, E.W.; Tierney, E.F.; Rios-Burrows, N.; Mokdad, A.H.; Ford, E.S.; et al. The evolving diabetes burden in the United States. *Ann. Intern. Med.* **2004**, *140*, 945–950. [CrossRef]

3. Lu, Y.; Wang, N.; Chen, Y.; Nie, X.; Li, Q.; Han, B.; Chen, Y.; Xia, F.; Cang, Z.; Lu, M.; et al. Health-related quality of life in type-2 diabetes patients: A cross-sectional study in East China. *BMC Endocr. Disord.* **2017**, *17*, 38. [CrossRef]
4. Fal, A.M.; Jankowska, B.; Uchmanowicz, I.; Sen, M.; Panaszek, B.; Polanski, J. Type 2 diabetes quality of life patients treated with insulin and oral hypoglycemic medication. *Acta Diabetol.* **2011**, *48*, 237–242. [CrossRef] [PubMed]
5. Scarpello, J. Improving survival with metformin: The evidence base today. *Diabetes Metab.* **2003**, *29*, 6S36–6S43. [CrossRef] [PubMed]
6. ElSayed, N.A.; Aleppo, G.; Aroda, V.R.; Bannuru, R.R.; Brown, F.M.; Bruemmer, D.; Collins, B.S.; Hilliard, M.E.; Isaacs, D.; Johnson, E.L.; et al. 9. Pharmacologic Approaches to Glycemic Treatment: Standards of Care in Diabetes-2023. *Diabetes Care* **2023**, *46* (Suppl. S1), S140–S157. [CrossRef]
7. Fang, M.; Wang, D.; Coresh, J.; Selvin, E. Trends in diabetes treatment and control in US adults, 1999–2018. *N. Engl. J. Med.* **2021**, *384*, 2219–2228. [CrossRef]
8. Le, P.; Chaitoff, A.; Misra-Hebert, A.D.; Ye, W.; Herman, W.H.; Rothberg, M.B. Use of antihyperglycemic medications in US adults: An analysis of the National Health and Nutrition Examination Survey. *Diabetes Care* **2020**, *43*, 1227–1233. [CrossRef]
9. Lo, K.B.; Gul, F.; Ram, P.; Kluger, A.Y.; Tecson, K.M.; McCullough, P.A.; Rangaswami, J. The effects of SGLT2 inhibitors on cardiovascular and renal outcomes in diabetic patients: A systematic review and meta-analysis. *Cardiorenal Med.* **2020**, *10*, 1–10. [CrossRef]
10. Cruz Rivera, S.; McMullan, C.; Jones, L.; Kyte, D.; Slade, A.; Calvert, M. The impact of patient-reported outcome data from clinical trials: Perspectives from international stakeholders. *J. Patient-Rep. Outcomes* **2020**, *4*, 51. [CrossRef]
11. Eliya, Y.; Averbuch, T.; Le, N.; Xie, F.; Thabane, L.; Mamas, M.A.; Van Spall, H.G.C. Temporal Trends and Factors Associated With the Inclusion of Patient-Reported Outcomes in Heart Failure Randomized Controlled Trials: A Systematic Review. *J. Am. Heart Assoc.* **2021**, *10*, e022353. [CrossRef]
12. Calvert, M.; Kyte, D.; Mercieca-Bebber, R.; Slade, A.; Chan, A.-W.; King, M.T.; The SPIRIT-PRO Group. Guidelines for inclusion of patient-reported outcomes in clinical trial protocols: The SPIRIT-PRO extension. *JAMA* **2018**, *319*, 483–494. [CrossRef]
13. Efficace, F.; Fayers, P.; Pusic, A.; Cemal, Y.; Yanagawa, J.; Jacobs, M.; la Sala, A.; Cafaro, V.; Whale, K.; Rees, J.; et al. Quality of patient-reported outcome reporting across cancer randomized controlled trials according to the CONSORT patient-reported outcome extension: A pooled analysis of 557 trials. *Cancer* **2015**, *121*, 3335–3342. [CrossRef] [PubMed]
14. Meraya, A.M.; Alwhaibi, M. Health related quality of life and healthcare utilization among adults with diabetes and kidney and eye complications in the United States. *Health Qual. Life Outcomes* **2020**, *18*, 85. [CrossRef] [PubMed]
15. Campbell, J.A.; Bishu, K.G.; Walker, R.J.; Egede, L.E. Trends of medical expenditures and quality of life in US adults with diabetes: The medical expenditure panel survey, 2002–2011. *Health Qual. Life Outcomes* **2017**, *15*, 70. [CrossRef] [PubMed]
16. Agency for Healthcare Research and Quality (AHRQb). Medical Expenditure Panel Survey, Survey Background. Available online: https://www.meps.ahrq.gov/mepsweb/about_meps/survey_back.jsp (accessed on 31 January 2023).
17. Kathe, N.; Hayes, C.J.; Bhandari, N.R.; Payakachat, N. Assessment of Reliability and Validity of SF-12v2 among a Diabetic Population. *Value Health* **2018**, *21*, 432–440. [CrossRef] [PubMed]
18. Ware, J.; Kosinski, M.; Keller, S. *How to Score the SF-12 Physical and Mental Health Summary Scales Boston*; The Health Institute: Springfield, MA, USA, 1995; p. 2.
19. Mouelhi, Y.; Jouve, E.; Castelli, C.; Gentile, S. How is the minimal clinically important difference established in health-related quality of life instruments? Review of anchors and methods. *Health Qual. Life Outcomes* **2020**, *18*, 136. [CrossRef] [PubMed]
20. Fu, V.; Weatherall, M.; McNaughton, H. Estimating the minimal clinically important difference for the Physical Component Summary of the Short Form 36 for patients with stroke. *J. Int. Med. Res.* **2021**, *49*, 03000605211067902. [CrossRef]
21. Jayadevappa, R.; Cook, R.; Chhatre, S. Minimal important difference to infer changes in health-related quality of life—A systematic review. *J. Clin. Epidemiol.* **2017**, *89*, 188–198. [CrossRef]
22. StataCorp. *Stata Statistical Software: Release 15*; StataCorp LLC: College Station, TX, USA, 2017.
23. Adami, G.; Gatti, D.; Rossini, M.; Orsolini, G.; Pollastri, F.; Bertoldo, E.; Viapiana, O.; Giollo, A.; Fassio, A. Risk of fragility fractures in obesity and diabetes: A retrospective analysis on a nation-wide cohort. *Osteoporos. Int.* **2020**, *31*, 2113–2122. [CrossRef]
24. Blonde, L.; Khunti, K.; Harris, S.B.; Meizinger, C.; Skolnik, N.S. Interpretation and impact of real-world clinical data for the practicing clinician. *Adv. Ther.* **2018**, *35*, 1763–1774. [CrossRef] [PubMed]
25. Mishra, R.; Krishan, S.; Siddiqui, A.N.; Kapur, P.; Khayyam, K.U.; Rai, P.K.; Sharma, M. Impact of metformin therapy on health-related quality of life outcomes in tuberculosis patients with diabetes mellitus in India: A prospective study. *Int. J. Clin. Pract.* **2021**, *75*, e13864. [CrossRef] [PubMed]
26. Basit, A. Assessing health related quality of life in diabetic subjects by SF 36 questionnaire in a tertiary care diabetes unit of Karachi, Pakistan. *Int. J. Adv. Res.* **2014**, *2*, 13–17.
27. Lau, C.-Y.; Qureshi, A.; Scott, S. Association between glycaemic control and quality of life in diabetes mellitus. *J. Postgrad. Med.* **2004**, *50*, 189. [PubMed]
28. Venkataraman, K.; Wee, H.; Leow, M.; Tai, E.; Lee, J.; Lim, S.; Tavintharan, S.; Wong, T.Y.; Ma, S.; Heng, D.; et al. Associations between complications and health-related quality of life in individuals with diabetes. *Clin. Endocrinol.* **2013**, *78*, 865–873. [CrossRef] [PubMed]

29. Rizza, S.; Cardellini, M.; Porzio, O.; Pecchioli, C.; Savo, A.; Cardolini, I.; Senese, N.; Lauro, D.; Sbraccia, P.; Lauro, R.; et al. Pioglitazone improves endothelial and adipose tissue dysfunction in pre-diabetic CAD subjects. *Atherosclerosis* **2011**, *215*, 180–183. [CrossRef]
30. Dormandy, J.A.; Charbonnel, B.; Eckland, D.J.; Erdmann, E.; Massi-Benedetti, M.; Moules, I.K.; Skene, A.M.; Tan, M.H.; Lefèbvre, P.J.; Murray, G.D.; et al. Secondary prevention of macrovascular events in patients with type 2 diabetes in the PROactive Study (PROspective pioglitAzone Clinical Trial In macroVascular Events): A randomised controlled trial. *Lancet* **2005**, *366*, 1279–1289. [CrossRef]
31. Tanne, J.H. FDA places "black box" warning on antidiabetes drugs. *BMJ* **2007**, *334*, 1237. [CrossRef]
32. Abdelmoneim, A.; Eurich, D.; Light, P.; Senior, P.; Seubert, J.; Makowsky, M.; Simpson, S.H. Cardiovascular safety of sulphonylureas: Over 40 years of continuous controversy without an answer. *Diabetes Obes. Metab.* **2015**, *17*, 523–532. [CrossRef]
33. Rizza, S.; Piciucchi, G.; Mavilio, M.; Longo, S.; Montagna, M.; Tatonetti, R.; Nucera, A.; Federici, M. Effect of deprescribing in elderly patients with type 2 diabetes: iDegLira might improve quality of life. *Biomed. Pharmacother.* **2021**, *144*, 112341. [CrossRef]
34. Russell-Jones, D.; Khan, R. Insulin-associated weight gain in diabetes-causes, effects and coping strategies. *Diabetes Obes. Metab.* **2007**, *9*, 799–812. [CrossRef] [PubMed]
35. Sola, D.; Rossi, L.; Schianca, G.P.C.; Maffioli, P.; Bigliocca, M.; Mella, R.; Corlianò, F.; Fra, G.P.; Bartoli, E.; Derosa, G. State of the art paper sulfonylureas and their use in clinical practice. *Arch. Med. Sci.* **2015**, *11*, 840–848. [CrossRef] [PubMed]
36. Stolar, M. Safety and efficacy of Pioglitazone/Metformin combination therapy in treatment of type 2 diabetes: A rationale for earlier use. *Clin. Med. Ther.* **2009**, *1*, CMT.S2370. [CrossRef]
37. Cai, X.-L.; Ji, L.-N. *Treatment Response between Asian and Non-Asian Patients with Type 2 Diabetes: Is There Any Similarity or Difference?* Chinese Medical Journals Publishing House Co., Ltd.: Beijing, China, 2019; pp. 1–3.
38. Poghosyan, H.; Stock, S.; Sheldon, L.K.; Cromwell, J.; Cooley, M.E.; Nerenz, D.R. Racial disparities in health-related quality of life after lung cancer surgery: Findings from the cancer care outcomes research and surveillance consortium. *J. Thorac. Oncol.* **2015**, *10*, 1404–1412. [CrossRef] [PubMed]
39. Velasco-Mondragon, E.; Jimenez, A.; Palladino-Davis, A.G.; Davis, D.; Escamilla-Cejudo, J.A. Hispanic health in the USA: A scoping review of the literature. *Public Health Rev.* **2016**, *37*, 31. [CrossRef] [PubMed]
40. Krawczyk-Suszek, M.; Kleinrok, A. Health-Related Quality of Life (HRQoL) of people over 65 years of age. *Int. J. Environ. Res. Public Health* **2022**, *19*, 625. [CrossRef]
41. Safieddine, B.; Sperlich, S.; Epping, J.; Lange, K.; Geyer, S. Development of comorbidities in type 2 diabetes between 2005 and 2017 using German claims data. *Sci. Rep.* **2021**, *11*, 11149. [CrossRef]
42. Goel, M.; Dhuldhule, S.; Prakash, A.; Ghotekar, L.H. Assessing health-related quality of life in patients with diabetes mellitus at a Tertiary Care Center in Central Delhi. *Indian J. Commun. Med. Off. Publ. Indian Assoc. Prev. Soc. Med.* **2019**, *44*, 171.
43. Aro, S.; Kangas, T.; Reunanen, A.; Salinto, M.; Koivisto, V. Hospital use among diabetic patients and the general population. *Diabetes Care* **1994**, *17*, 1320–1329. [CrossRef]
44. Comino, E.J.; Harris, M.F.; Islam, M.; Tran, D.T.; Jalaludin, B.; Jorm, L.; Flack, J.; Haas, M. Impact of diabetes on hospital admission and length of stay among a general population aged 45 year or more: A record linkage study. *BMC Health Serv. Res.* **2015**, *15*, 12. [CrossRef]
45. Donnan, P.T.; Leese, G.P.; Morris, A.D.; Audit, D. Research in Tayside SMMUC. Hospitalizations for people with type 1 and type 2 diabetes compared with the nondiabetic population of Tayside, Scotland: A retrospective cohort study of resource use. *Diabetes Care* **2000**, *23*, 1774–1779. [CrossRef] [PubMed]
46. Hall, M.J.; Rui, P.; Schwartzman, A. *Emergency Department Visits by Patients Aged 45 and over with Diabetes: United States, 2015*; NCHS Data Brief, no 301; National Center for Health Statistics: Hyattsville, MD, USA, 2018.
47. Mamo, Y.; Bekele, F.; Nigussie, T.; Zewudie, A. Determinants of poor glycemic control among adult patients with type 2 diabetes mellitus in Jimma University Medical Center, Jimma zone, south west Ethiopia: A case control study. *BMC Endocr. Disord.* **2019**, *19*, 91. [CrossRef] [PubMed]
48. Bolen, S.; Feldman, L.; Vassy, J.; Wilson, L.; Yeh, H.-C.; Marinopoulos, S.; Wiley, C.; Selvin, E.; Wilson, R.; Bass, E.; et al. Systematic review: Comparative effectiveness and safety of oral medications for type 2 diabetes mellitus. *Ann. Intern. Med.* **2007**, *147*, 386–399. [CrossRef]
49. Roumie, C.L.; Hung, A.M.; Greevy, R.A.; Grijalva, C.G.; Liu, X.; Murff, H.J.; Elasy, T.A.; Griffin, M.R. Comparative effectiveness of sulfonylurea and metformin monotherapy on cardiovascular events in type 2 diabetes mellitus: A cohort study. *Ann. Intern. Med.* **2012**, *157*, 601–610. [CrossRef] [PubMed]
50. Lipscombe, L.L.; Gomes, T.; Lévesque, L.E.; Hux, J.E.; Juurlink, D.N.; Alter, D.A. Thiazolidinediones and cardiovascular outcomes in older patients with diabetes. *JAMA* **2007**, *298*, 2634–2643. [CrossRef]
51. Landon, B.E.; Zaslavsky, A.M.; Souza, J.; Ayanian, J.Z. Use of diabetes medications in traditional Medicare and Medicare Advantage. *Am. J. Manag. Care* **2021**, *27*, e80.

healthcare

MDPI

Article

Analysis of Costs Associated with the Use of Personalized Automated Dosing Systems versus Manual Preparation in a Residential Center for the Elderly in Extremadura

Mª del Carmen Lozano-Estevan [1], Liliana Guadalupe González-Rodríguez [1], Rafael Lozano-Fernández [2], Jorge Velázquez-Saornil [3,*], José Luis Sánchez-Manzano [4], Iván Herrera-Peco [5], José Antonio Guerra-Guirao [6] and Pilar Leal-Carbajo [7]

1 VALORNUT Research Group, Department of Nutrition and Food Science, Faculty of Pharmacy, Complutense University of Madrid, 28040 Madrid, Spain
2 Departamento de Química en Ciencias Farmacéuticas, Facultad de Farmacia, Universidad Complutense de Madrid, 28040 Madrid, Spain
3 NEUMUSK Research Group, Departamento de Fisioterapia, Facultad de Ciencias de la Salud, Universidad Católica de Ávila, 05005 Ávila, Spain
4 Farmacia Comunitaria de Cáceres, 10001 Cáceres, Spain
5 Faculty of Health Sciences, Alfonso X el Sabio University, Avda. Universidad, 1, Villanueva de la Cañada, 28691 Madrid, Spain
6 Departamento de Farmacología, Farmacognosia y Botánica, Facultad de Farmacia, Universidad Complutense de Madrid, 28040 Madrid, Spain
7 Servicio de Farmacia, Centro de Salud del Servicio Extremeño de Salud La Roca de la Sierra, 06070 Badajoz, Spain
* Correspondence: jorge.velazquezsaornil@ucavila.es; Tel.: +34-920-251-020

Abstract: Introduction: During the SARS-CoV-2 pandemic, there has been a decrease in the supervision of the medication of subjects with chronic diseases. Customized automated dosing systems (SPDA) are devices that allow medication to be dispensed and administered, which have proven to be safe and effective for the patient and cost-effective for the healthcare system. Methods: an intervention study was carried out on patients from January to December 2019 in a residential centre for the elderly with more than 100 beds. The economic costs derived from manual dosing were compared with those of an automated preparation (Robotik Technology®). Results: Of the 198 patients included, 195 (97.47%) of them were polymedicated. Of the total of 276 active substances of registered medicinal products, it was possible to include them in the process of automating the preparation of the SPDA 105 active pharmaceutical ingredients. A cost reduction of EUR 5062.39 per year was found using SPDA. Taking into account the active ingredients of emblistable and non-emblistable medicines, the use of SPDA resulted in savings of EUR 6120.40 per year. The system contributed to the detection of cases of therapeutic duplication and reduced the time to prepare the medication. Conclusions: the use of SPDA is a useful and economically profitable strategy for its use in residential centres for the elderly.

Keywords: administration; dosage; polypharmacy; cost-analysis

check for updates

Citation: Lozano-Estevan, M.d.C.; González-Rodríguez, L.G.; Lozano-Fernández, R.; Velázquez-Saornil, J.; Sánchez-Manzano, J.L.; Herrera-Peco, I.; Guerra-Guirao, J.A.; Leal-Carbajo, P. Analysis of Costs Associated with the Use of Personalized Automated Dosing Systems versus Manual Preparation in a Residential Center for the Elderly in Extremadura. *Healthcare* **2023**, *11*, 620. https://doi.org/10.3390/healthcare11040620

Academic Editor: Georges Adunlin

Received: 20 December 2022
Revised: 3 February 2023
Accepted: 16 February 2023
Published: 19 February 2023

1. Introduction

In the SARS-CoV-2 pandemic situation, the need to improve the continuity of care and ensure access to medicines in a safe and efficient manner became evident [1–4]. The pandemic has greatly affected the care of chronic pathologies [5,6]. In the case of polymedicated, non-institutionalised patients with multiple pathologies, there is also a decrease in the supervision of medication by relatives or direct caregivers, as visits have been reduced due to periods of restricted mobility [5,7].

The model of personalized, integrated pharmaceutical care becomes more relevant in this pandemic context [8–10], giving greater importance to the role of the community pharmacist after the act of dispensing medicines, participating in the administration of medicines with tools such as personalised dosage systems (PDS) that allow the medication to be organised using special blister packs, on set days and at set times. SPDs are an aid to pharmaceutical care integrated into the continuity of care for polymedicated patients while ensuring better adherence to the pharmacological treatment of these polymedicated patients and, therefore, saving the health system money by avoiding therapeutic non-compliance and admissions due to medication errors [11–14].

The patient receives his or her medication organised in a personalised system, which improves adherence to treatment, thereby optimising the control of consumption as it allows for the safekeeping of the remaining medication not dispensed at the pharmacy [15]. At the same time, it helps polymedicated patients to maintain their independence and safety and improves the quality of care and the efficiency and sustainability of the healthcare system [16–18].

In a residential care home for the elderly, patients have multiple pathologies and the average consumption of medicines is higher than for those who continue to live at home [18]. The manual administration of these medications is a common practice in residential centres without the intervention of the community pharmacist, and this practice has repercussions on patient safety because it is associated with dosage errors, non-compliance with dosage, incorrect interpretation of medical indications and lack of organisation of inventories [9]. In response to this, the use of personalised dosing systems (PDS) performed by community pharmacists in the Pharmacy Office has been proposed. Personalised dispensing systems can be prepared by the pharmacist manually or automatically by a blister robot, and in this case, we are talking about personalised dispensing automation systems (PDA). These robotic blistering systems constitute a new technology capable of reducing the time required for the preparation and distribution of medicines in individualised doses.

In general, only solid oral preparations with good physical, chemical and pharmaceutical stability are suitable for inclusion in SPDs, provided that they are stable outside the original primary packaging at room temperature for the period of unblistering, preparation, delivery and use. Non-oral dosage forms, such as ova or suppositories, and non-solid oral dosage forms, such as sachets, should be excluded from SPD. Thermolabile (refrigerator storage between 2 and 8 °C) medicinal products should also be excluded [18].

Extremadura has a population that is older and more dependent than the national average and usually resides in rural areas [19]. This has been associated with the implementation of both public and private resources to improve the care of the adult population residing in residential centres or day centres [20]. In order to overcome deficiencies in the supply and dispensation of medicines, the use of SPDA in these facilities has been proposed [21,22]. However, it is not known to what extent these systems are associated with a reduction in financial expenditure. For this reason, the main objective of this study is to compare the costs of manual drug administration with SPDA. Performed by pharmacists in a Pharmacy Office in a residential center for the elderly in Extremadura.

2. Materials and Methods

An intervention study was carried out in which a model of pharmaceutical care integrated into the care model of the resident population of the Ciudad Jardín Residential Centre in Caceres was designed as the object of study, using personalised automated dosage systems (SPDA).

This study was carried out from January to December 2018 and January to December 2019 on a closed multi-pathological and elderly population in the Ciudad Jardín residential centre, with a private management model and a mixed public–private medication supply system of the Extremadura Health Service/Pharmacy Office. As it is a residential centre of more than 100 beds, part of the supply of medicines for patients is provided by the Hospital Pharmacy of the referral hospital and the medicines that the hospital does not have in stock are supplied by a Pharmacy Office.

This residential centre places fortnightly orders for medicines from the Hospital Pharmacy of the Hospital San Pedro de Alcántara according to the patient's treatment schedule for 15 days. Residential centre does not have any medicine management programme to order the exact consumption of medicines to be consumed in the next 15 days, so the nurses make an estimate according to the existing stock and with reference to previous orders accumulating in the residential centre to create a large stock of medicines. The Ciudad Jardín Residential Centre has 240 beds. The two groups of patients, both in 2018 and 2019, were made up of the same patients in order to avoid selection bias.

During 2018, the Garden City Residential Centre used the manual pill dispenser method by the staff. Starting in 2019, throughout the year, the production of SPDA blister packs using the medicine blistering robot (RobotikTechnology®) was introduced at the Pilar Leal Pharmacy in Alcuéscar, Spain.

Pharmaceutical dosage forms that can be included in both manual and automated personalised drug delivery systems include only solid oral medicinal products with good physical, chemical and pharmaceutical stability, provided that they are stable outside the original primary packaging at room temperature for the period covering unblistering, preparation, delivery and use. Non-oral dosage forms, such as ova or suppositories, and non-solid oral dosage forms, such as so-bres, should be excluded from SPD. Thermolabile (refrigerator storage between 2 and 8 °C) medicinal products should also be excluded.

This modification in the way medication is administered was used to compare the costs of manual and automated production (year 2018 compared to 2019). The medication supply system was the same in both 2018 and 2019. The Garden City Residential Centre has a supply of public and private medication. Public management corresponds to the Extremadura Health System, and the private management corresponds to the Pharmacy Office.

In order to implement the model, project management techniques, process management, training for the people involved in the process and a study to assess the previous situation in terms of financial and patient safety were used in the different phases of the project's implementation.

A homogeneous population was considered in terms of the main variables: age over 64 years of age and without a direct reference person for medication management. The following variables were chosen as study variables: age, gender, co-payment of the individual health card (IHC), pharmaceutical expenditure on medicines, medical devices and medicines not financed supplied by the Extremadura Health Service and patient co-payment at the Alcuéscar Pharmacy Office. The number of medicines consumed by each patient was also taken into account, and polymedication was considered to be the consumption of three or more medicines/per day.

The information was obtained from the electronic and paper prescriptions from the geriatric centre's doctor, as well as from the orders for medicines received at the Residential Centre from the Hospital Pharmacy of the San Pedro de Alcántara Hospital in Cáceres. Data on the consumption of medicines were also obtained from the management software "Farmadosis" AMCO+ (FARMADOSIS S.L., Palma de Mallorca, Spain), a management programme used by the Pharmacy Office for the weekly production of SPDA medication that connects the SPDA robot with healthcare professionals of the residential centre, as well as with the technology and information systems necessary to coordinate the pharmaceutical care with healthcare professionals in the nursing of this centre. The Pharmacy Office carries out the weekly emblisting of patients' medication for production with the SPDA system, which makes it possible to obtain metrics related to medication consumption.

All patients of this centre who agreed to participate were included in a consecutive selection process. For this purpose, the patients were given an informed consent form explaining the study in detail and that the data obtained would be anonymous and would only be used for the purpose of the study.

The inclusion criteria were as follows:

- Persons with a stay of 30 days or more at the Ciudad Jardín Residence.
- A user of 1 or more drugs for a period greater than or equal to 30 consecutive days of chronic medication.
- Absence of a direct primary caregiver.
- Sign the authorisation and informed consent included in the standard work protocol (SOP) of the SPDA of the Pharmacy Office in order to relocate their medication to the SPDA's list at the Alcuéscar Pharmacy Office.
- To have their treatments financed by the Extremadura Health System (SES), with TSI 001, 002, 003, 004 and 005, as established by Royal Decree-Law 16/2012, of 20 April, on urgent measures to guarantee the sustainability of the National Health System and improve the quality and safety of its services [23].

The exclusion criteria were as follows:

- Stay of less than 30 days (either due to change of residence or death before 30 days).
- Non-user of medicines.
- Not signing the informed consent form.
- Belonging to companies or mutual insurance companies

Discontinued medications were excluded for patients with chronic medications.

The model was subject to continuous quality assessment, with measures adapted to the needs and lines identified as possible improvements.

In September 2018, the situation analysis phase was carried out prior to the implementation of the pharmaceutical care model in the residential centre. Meetings were held with healthcare staff, especially for reviewing the processes related to patient treatment. A working methodology adapted to what they were doing was proposed so that the implementation of personalised pharmaceutical care could be integrated into the usual working system. The healthcare staff of the residential centre, responsible for administering medicines to patients, were trained in SPD systems for medicines to ensure patient safety and without extensive modification of routine clinical practice.

We retrieved data on medications consumed by patients throughout 2018 and demographic data on all patients discharged from the centre. They were segmented by age, gender and type of health coverage. Training of healthcare staff was intensified for the implementation of this new model.

To this end, the technology and information systems in place were used to coordinate pharmaceutical care with the healthcare professionals at the residential centre.

During the period analysed, in 2018 and 2019, a total of 198 patients who met the inclusion criteria for the study were included each year.

The expenditure associated with the manual dosing of the residential center in manual devices was quantified and compared with the expenditure associated with the elaboration of the SPDA made by the Pilar Leal Carbajo Community Pharmacy Office.

The efficiency of personnel and material resources was analysed. At all times, the preparation of active ingredients of medicines was ensured through the SPDA. Qualified and duly certified staff came from the community Pharmacy Office of Pilar Leal Carbajo.

The time spent by healthcare staff at the residential centre who prepared the individual pill dispensers with medicines using the manual method in 2018 was analysed, along with the associated economic expenditure, which was compared with the preparation of medication using the SPDAs in the Pharmacy Office in 2019 and its associated economic expenditure.

3. Results

Patients included in the study who met the inclusion criteria were 198 patients in each study year.

3.1. Results Regarding Polymedication:

The proportion of polymedicated patients in the study population was 97.47% of the total number of patients with any medication. When analysing the polypharmacy of the population, it was observed that only five patients had less than three drugs.

A total of 276 active pharmaceutical ingredients consumed each year by the patients included in the study were recorded. Of these, 99 active pharmaceutical ingredients were found that could not be reblistered due to their pharmaceutical form in the SPDA and were administered manually by the healthcare staff at the healthcare centre. The remaining 177 active ingredients of medicines consumed each year by the patients included in the study could be reblistered in the SPDA robot prepared in the Pharmacy Office. Of these 177, 72 active ingredients of medicines were supplied by the community Pharmacy Office through medical prescriptions, and the remaining 105 active ingredients of medicines were supplied by the Extremadura Health Service to the Ciudad Jardín residential centre.

3.2. Results Relating to the Expenditure Obtained for the Medication Administered by SPDA:

When analysing the data on essential medicines provided by San Pedro de Alcántara Hospital to the residential centre, a decrease in the number of units of medicines requested from the hospital by means of fortnightly orders by the residential centre was observed in 2019 compared to 2018.

The number of units of medicines provided by San Pedro de Alcántara Hospital and spent in 2019 when using the SPDA is 330,271 U (with an associated expenditure of EUR 83,374.90) compared to 2018 which resulted in 381,740 U (with an associated expenditure of EUR 88,437.29). This reduction in expenditure using the system proposed in this study was EUR 5062.39 per year.

The overall consumption of medicines (essential and non-essential) was analysed using the integrated pharmaceutical care system with SPDA: it was observed that in the model presented, a total of 452,997 units of medicines were consumed in 2018 at the cost of EUR 178,745.74. This compares to 2019, when 402,638 units of medicines were consumed with a PVP ii cost of EUR 172,625.34.

This represents a saving of EUR 6120.40, but this model has not had a significant influence on the decrease in the number of units of non-emblistable medicines.

This study did not quantify the medication changes that occurred from one year to the next (2018 to 2019) in patients, so this decrease can be partly can be associated with this fact. What was reduced was the overstocking of medicines in the residential centre by ordering medicines without precision in quantity, avoiding future expiry of these medicines.

The proposed system contributed to the detection of two cases of therapeutic duplicity, i.e., the presence of two medicines of the same therapeutic class, one of which was duplicity of analgesics and one was duplicity of analgesics; the patient had been prescribed paracetamol one gram and the combination tramadol/paracetamol 37.5 mg/325 mg, another was duplicity of anti-ulcer drugs, the patient had omeprazole 40 mg and esomeprazole 20 mg. An alert record sheet was created for the nursing staff, who systematically checked the patient's visual check by them prior to the administration of medication, and reported the subjective perception of more cases where they self-corrected the duplicity error but did not record it prior to the implementation of the integrated pharmaceutical care model.

The study population comprised 46 men and 152 women. Nine patients were younger than 65 years, 40 patients between 65 and 80 years and 149 patients older than 80 years.

According to the classification established by the Ministry of Health, with regard to the TSI assigned, we see that 186 residents out of the 198 total have a TSI002, 93.93% of the total.

After analysing all the data according to the TSI of the patients in the residential centre, the only TSI to be considered is TSI001, TSI002 and TSI003, as no results were obtained for the rest as there were no patients in this range. From TSI001, a total of eight users were obtained for consideration. TSI002 yielded 186 users, of which 4 had a co-payment ceiling of 18.52 euros, leaving 182 residents with a co-payment ceiling of 8.23 euros for medicines.

Finally, from TSI003, there was only one user who paid 40% of the cost of his medication. The data on the medicines financed and the co-payments made by patients with TSI002 were included, as well as the co-payments that patients would make if the supply were managed entirely by the pharmacy that serves the geriatric centre, instead of being shared with the Extremadura Health Service.

In the Ciudad Jardín Residential Centre, there is a shared supply between the Extremadura Health Service and the Pharmacy Office of Alcuéscar. It was observed that the pharmaceutical co-payment expenditure was lower than that which each resident should have to pay for the prescribed treatments. This is usually the case in residential centres in Extremadura with less than 100 beds; it is the user who finances this expense and not the Extremadura Health Service, according to the agreement between the Pharmaceutical Association of Cáceres and the Extremadura Health Service [3].

On analysing the consumption generated by the patients of the Ciudad Jardín Residential Centre, a deviation of pharmaceutical products non-financed pharmaceutical products supplied from the Pharmacy Department of the San Pedro de Alcántara Hospital in Cáceres. This justifies a separate quantitative analysis of the amount at PVL ii and PVP ii according to Botplus as of 2018 [24] and the number of units served during the year. These medicines are financed for patients who are in facilities with more than 100 beds but not for patients residing in their own homes or in facilities with less than 100 beds, as currently established.

In other words, in order to dispense these medicines, the Extremadura Health Service buys them at the LMP, so an expenditure of EUR 18,888.11 is imputed. However, if these same patients were to reside in their own homes or in a residential centre with fewer than 100 beds, this cost would not be borne by the Extremadura Health Service but would be financed by the patient themself, regardless of the patient's other socio-economic variables.

This agreement creates a situation in which residents in centres with more than 100 beds would have a saving of EUR 28,119.46 and the Extremadura health service would have an expense of EUR 18,888.11.

Individual medication preparation time was accounted for both with the SPDA (2019) and manual preparation of weekly pill dispensers (2018). Both processes were carried out with two pharmacists for SPDA preparation and three nurses for the manual preparation of pill dispensers, who were familiar with each of the preparation processes. Average preparation time and human resource expenditure were calculated. The analysed expenditure for the manual preparation of weekly medication for 240 residents is shown in Tables 1 and 2.

Table 1. Patients included in the study with polypharmacy.

Number of Medicines	Patients (*N = 198*)
1	1
2	4
3	8
4	22
5	25
6	26
7	34
8	26
9	23
10	8
11	9
12	8
13	1
14	3
Total patients	198

Table 2. Economic study for the manual preparation of weekly pill dispensers for 240 residents of the Ciudad Jardín centre.

Manual preparation time of 1 Pillbox per week with 4 intakes per day	14–15 min/pill dispenser
Number of pill dispensers per month	4.33 units (average for 52 weeks per year)
Total preparation time for one month for one patient	64.95 min/month/patient 1.08 h/month/patient
Cost of salary + social insurance of nursing personnel	12.18 EUR/h (according to agreement)
Cost of manual pill dispenser preparation per patient	1.08 h/month/patient × 12.18 EUR/h = 13.15 EUR/month/patient Miscellaneous maintenance costs: 0.80 EUR/patient/month
Costs of consumables and supplies to be borne by the Geriatric Centre	Pill dispenser renewal: 35 EUR/unit (10% annual renewal) Annual medication trolleys: 1.500 EUR/unit (one unit every 3 years) Cleaning products, gloves: 30 EUR/month
Costs of consumables and supplies to be borne by the Geriatric Centre	13.95/month/patient × 240 patients = 3348 EUR/month for 240 patients

The cost of producing SPDA blister packs of medicines was also analysed. The costs of consumables are borne by the Pharmacy Office, which was cost-efficient for the health system, as well as all costs of supplies, personnel and legislative requirements. The expenditure analysed for automated SPDA preparation of weekly medication for 240 patients of the residential centre is shown in Table 3.

Table 3. Economic study for the automated preparation of weekly SPDA for 240 patients of the residential centre Ciudad Jardín.

Manual preparation time of 1 SPDA per week with 4 intakes per day	1 min/patient/28 sachets
Number of SPDA per month	120 sachets (average for the 52 weeks with medication changes during the month)
Total preparation time for one month for one patient	1 min/month/patient 0.066 h/month/patient
Cost of salary + S.S. of pharmaceutical personnel	16.83 EUR/h (according to agreement)
SPDA preparation cost per patient	0.066 h/month/patient × 16.83 EUR/hour = 1.11 EUR/month/patient 0.03 EUR/bag × 120 bags/month/patient/patient = 3.60 EUR/month/patient Other expenses attributable to the O.F. = 1.28 EUR/month/patient
Costs of consumables and supplies to be borne by the F.O.	Ink ribbon and pouch film: 120 EUR/4.000 pouches produced (0.03 EUR/bag)
	Technology investments and monthly software maintenance: 150 EUR/month
	Electricity, insurance and equipment: 30 EUR/month
Total SPDA preparation for 240 patients	5.99/month/patient × 240 patients = 1437.60 EUR/month for 240 patients assumed by the Pharmacy Office of Alcuéscar

The SPDA was faster in the preparation of a patient's monthly medication than the manual procedure that has been used to the current time. On the basis of these working times, the total cost was estimated: a total cost of EUR 3348 per medication preparation process per month for 240 patients in 2018 (manual system) and a total expenditure in 2019 (with SPDA) of EUR 1437.6 for 240 patients.

At the time of the study, as the SES supplies the user without strict control, it receives EUR 5978.30 less and has an expenditure of EUR 18,888.11. In the study, the SES has a total loss of EUR 24,866.41 (EUR 5978.30 + EUR 18,888.11). In addition to showing a difference in access to medication between residents in centres with more than 100 or less than 100 beds or at home, regardless of the socio-economic situation of each patient.

4. Discussion

The implementation of this model of personalised pharmaceutical care integrated into the care of institutionalised patients in the population studied shows an economic impact on both the Extremadura Health Service and the Ciudad Jardín Residential Centre. As it is included in comprehensive pharmaceutical care, with appropriate information systems, the model presented allows for the detection of duplicity and other medication errors and solving them in real-time [11,24,25]. This means improving the quality of patient prescribing and, therefore, patient compliance, contributing to the optimal control of chronic diseases in terms of medication management [26]. The professionalisation of medication supply and the presence of a pharmacist to review and monitor treatments, duplications and interactions on a personalised basis for each patient has been shown to contribute to the rationalisation of healthcare expenditure.

Non-financed medicines were quantified at PVL ii because this is the purchase price of these products, according to Botplus, as of 2018 [27]. This potentially represents a direct saving for the Extremadura Health Service in pharmaceutical expenditure for these patients in one year of using this personalised pharmaceutical care model [18]. As a cost-saving measure for the Extremadura Health System, by ceasing to request fortnightly bulk orders, non-financed medicines and medical devices would change the financer by being to be charged to the patient in centres with more than 100 beds [17]. Until now, in facilities with less than 100 beds or residents at home, this expenditure is charged to the user.

The residential centre that was under this system would have more hours per month of qualified health personnel to reassign to other occupations that would improve the quality of the centre and its patients, saving time in storage and placement of medicines and checking expiry dates, as well as saving money on the purchase of medication trolleys and their maintenance.

The pharmacy that participates in the pharmaceutical care of this model, which was implemented in the Ciudad Jardín residential centre, assumed direct investment costs in technology and information systems to carry out the SPDA of medicines, consumable materials necessary for weekly production, and the relevant legal obligations. Likewise, the hiring of personnel to provide a quality service to the residential centres is financially compensated by the profit margin on the increase in sales of the medicines and medical devices discussed during this study.

It is therefore important to consider this model of integrated pharmaceutical care in residential centres as an alternative to the current model in order to guarantee the sustainability of social and healthcare services while at the same time providing quality, patient safety and equity.

A more extensive study on equity of access to medication for patients living in facilities with less than 100 beds and no and not institutionalized would be needed [28].

One of the limitations of the study is that it focuses on a single centre and takes as a reference the medication control system of the residents of a single centre. However, it would be useful to extrapolate this system to other centres, so we believe that future research can be based on our work in order to contribute more scientific quality to the community. To date, there is no article that discusses this process of cost analysis associated with personalised dosing systems, comparing the two possibilities: manual versus automated preparation.

5. Conclusions

SPDAs are effective tools to optimise the pharmacological treatment of institutionalised elderly people and are safer and less costly than manual dosing of medicines. Their implementation in facilities has a positive economic impact on health services, as well as a way of incorporating integrated pharmaceutical care.

Author Contributions: Conceptualization, P.L.-C. and J.L.S.-M.; methodology, I.H.-P. and J.A.G.-G.; software, R.L.-F.; validation, P.L.-C., J.L.S.-M. and I.H.-P.; formal analysis, R.L.-F.; investigation, P.L.-C.; resources, J.V.-S.; data curation, L.G.G.-R.; writing—original draft preparation, J.V.-S.; writing—review and editing, J.V.-S. and P.L.-C.; visualization, L.G.G.-R. and I.H.-P.; supervision, M.d.C.L.-E.; project administration, M.d.C.L.-E.; funding acquisition, P.L.-C. and J.L.S.-M. All authors have read and agreed to the published version of the manuscript.

Funding: This research received no external funding.

Institutional Review Board Statement: Not applicable.

Informed Consent Statement: Informed consent was obtained from all subjects involved in the study. Written informed consent has been obtained from the patients to publish this paper.

Acknowledgments: We would like to thank the workers and managers of the Ciudad Jardín residential centre for their involvement in this research work.

Conflicts of Interest: The authors declare no conflict of interest.

References

1. Basu, S. Non-Communicable Disease Management in Vulnerable Patients during COVID-19. *Indian J. Med. Ethics* **2020**, *5*, 103–105. [CrossRef] [PubMed]
2. Fusco, A.; Dicuonzo, G.; Dell'Atti, V.; Tatullo, M. Blockchain in Healthcare: Insights on COVID-19. *Int. J. Environ. Res. Public Health* **2020**, *17*, 7167. [CrossRef] [PubMed]
3. Lakhani, M.; Lakhani, S.; Lakhani, P. Reimagining Healthcare after COVID-19: A New Normal for Medicine. *BMJ* **2020**, *369*, m2220. [CrossRef] [PubMed]
4. Masroor, S. Collateral Damage of COVID-19 Pandemic: Delayed Medical Care. *J. Card. Surg.* **2020**, *35*, 1345–1347. [CrossRef] [PubMed]
5. Zupanets, I.; Dobrova, V.; O Shilkina, O. Development of Theoretical Approaches to Pharmaceutical Care Improvement Considering the Modern Requirements of Health-Care System in Ukraine. *Asian J. Pharm. Clin. Res.* **2018**, *11*, 356. [CrossRef]
6. Abdo-Francis, J.M.; Bosques-Padilla, F.J.; Gutiérrez-Castrellon, P.; Sobrino-Cossío, S.R. El Daño Colateral de La Atención de La Pandemia de COVID-19. *Cirugía Y Cir.* **2020**, *88*, 799–804. [CrossRef] [PubMed]
7. Lesende, I.M. Lecciones Aprendidas Durante La Pandemia COVID-19 Sobre El Seguimiento de Pacientes Crónicos. *Atención Primaria* **2021**, *53*, 102180. [CrossRef] [PubMed]
8. Puchi-Gómez, C.; Paravic-Klijn, T.; Salazar, A. Indicadores de Calidad de La Atención En Salud En Hospitalización Domiciliaria: Revisión Integradora. *Aquichan* **2018**, *18*, 186–197. [CrossRef]
9. Farmacia. Ministerio de Sanidad, Servicios Sociales e Igualdad—Profesionales—Información al Consumidor. 2019. Available online: https://www.mscbs.gob.es/profesionales/farmacia/consenso/consenso.htm (accessed on 6 December 2022).
10. Pinzón Pulido, S.; Ferrer López, I.; Cáceres Fernández-Bolaños, R.; Hidalgo Fort, E.; Muñoz Chavero, F.; Navarro Matillas, B.; Rodríguez Gómez, S.; Espinosa Almendro, J.M.; Escudero Espinosa, C.; Patrocinio Polo, R.; et al. Más Allá Del COVID-19. Diseño de Un Nuevo Modelo de Atención Compartida Entre Farmacia Comunitaria y Atención Primaria. *Pharm. Care España* **2020**, *22*, 400–420.
11. Serra-Prat, M.; Regué, M.B.; Novellas, B.F.; Maragall, C.A. Eficacia de Un Sistema Personalizado de Dosificación (SPD) En La Mejoría Del Cumplimiento Terapéutico En Ancianos Polimedicados. *Atención Primaria* **2006**, *37*, 524–526. [CrossRef] [PubMed]
12. Arco, J.d.; Jesus, N.; de Buruaga, S.S. Sistemas Personalizados de Dosificación. Funcionamiento. *Farm. Prof.* **2008**, *22*, 36–40.
13. Hernández, E.L. Mariño. Sistemas Personalizados de Dosificación: Una Herramienta Para La Práctica Profesional Sanitaria En La Atención Farmacéutica. *Pharm. Care España* **2011**, *13*, 30.
14. Ruiz Loscertales, H. Los Sistemas Personalizados de Dosificación y Su Aportación a La Seguridad de Los Pacientes. 2017. Available online: http://hdl.handle.net/2445/114303 (accessed on 6 December 2022).
15. Olivas, N.J.; Majada, A.C.; Ochoa, M.D.P.H.; Valverde, A.M.; Rodríguez, M.L.M.; García, C.M. Sistemas Personalizados de Dosificación En Atención Primaria: Un Estudio Multidisciplinar. *Farm. Comunitarios* **2018**, *11*, 5–12. [CrossRef]

16. Merencio, E.; Jané, I.; Busquets, A.; Mestres, C.; Burniol, M.; Tous, S.; Iracheta, M.; Dellonder, N.; Mundet, M. Papel Del Farmacéutico Comunitario En La Quinta y Sexta Ola de La Pandemia de SARS-Cov2 En Cataluña. *Farm. Comunitarios* **2022**, *14*, 226. [CrossRef]
17. Agencia Española de Medicamentos y Productos Sanitarios. Buenas Prácticas de Distribución de Medicamentos de Uso Humano y Veterinario. 2019. Available online: https://www.aemps.gob.es/industria-farmaceutica/distribucion-farmaceutica/industria_distribucion_medicamentos_bpd_ue/ (accessed on 6 December 2022).
18. Jung, N.A.; Javier, A.M.; José, A.H. *Gasto Sanitario y Envejecimiento de La Población En España;* Documentos de Trabajo (Fundación BBVA): Bilbao, Spain, 2003.
19. Nieto, E.C. Manufacturing and Automation. *Ing. E Investig.* **2006**, *26*, 120–128. [CrossRef]
20. Sistema Nacional de Salud. Ministerio de Sanidad, Consumo y Bienestar Social—Organización Institucional. 2012. Available online: https://www.sanidad.gob.es/organizacion/sns/libroSNS.htm (accessed on 6 December 2022).
21. Jefatura de Estado. BOE.Es—BOE-A-2012-5403 Real Decreto-Ley 16/2012, de 20 de Abril, de Medidas Urgentes Para Garantizar La Sostenibilidad Del Sistema Nacional de Salud y Mejorar La Calidad y Seguridad de Sus Prestaciones. 2012. Available online: https://www.boe.es/buscar/act.php?id=BOE-A-2012-5403 (accessed on 6 December 2022).
22. Consejo General de Colegios Farmacéuticos. Buenas Prácticas En Farmacia Comunitaria. 2021. Available online: https://www.farmaceuticos.com/farmaceuticos/farmacia/buenas-practicas/buenas-practicas-en-farmacia-comunitaria/ (accessed on 6 December 2022).
23. Ley de Garantías y Uso Racional de Medicamentos y Productos Sanitarios: Impacto Económico. *Farm. Prof.* **2006**, *20*, 10–16.
24. Dupotey Varela, N.M.; Sedeño Argilagos, C.; Ramalho de Oliveira, D.; Rojas Vázquez, E.I.; Fernández Sánchez, E.; Reyes Hernández, I.; León Caballero, Y.; Lefevre, F.; Cavalcanti Lefevre, A.M. El Enfoque Holístico En La Atención Farmacéutica: Servicios de Gestión Integral de La Farmacoterapia. *Rev. Mex. De Cienc. Farm.* **2017**, *48*, 28–42.
25. Hernández, A.B.M.; Valdivieso, M.G.; Arasa, J.; Pintor, E.L. Estudio de Revisión de Las Ventajas e Inconvenientes de Los Sistemas Personalizados de Dosificación (SPD) y Evaluación de Su Adecuación al Perfil Del Paciente y Tipo de Farmacia. *FarmaJournal* **2020**, *5*, 47–54. [CrossRef]
26. Lenssen, R.K.; Schmitz, C.; Griesel, A.; Heidenreich, J.B.; Schulz, C.; Trautwein, N.; Marx, C.; Fitzner, U. Jaehde, and A. Eisert. Comprehensive Pharmaceutical Care to Prevent Drug-Related Readmissions of Dependent-Living Elderly Patients: A Randomized Controlled Trial. *BMC Geriatr.* **2018**, *18*, 135. [CrossRef] [PubMed]
27. De la Riva, J. Ebook XXIV Congreso AGE. 2023. Available online: http://congresoage.unizar.es/eBook/ (accessed on 6 December 2022).
28. de los Santos, F.R.; Valverde, P.R.; Rodríguez, C.M.; García, M.H. Análisis Del Modelo Salutogénico En España: Aplicación En Salud Pública e Implicaciones Para El Modelo de Activos En Salud. *Rev. Española Salud Pública* **2011**, *85*, 129–139. [CrossRef] [PubMed]

healthcare MDPI

Article

Barriers to Medication Review Process Implementation—Cross-Sectional Study among Community Pharmacists in Jordan

Mohammad Abu Assab *, Hamza Alhamad, Inas Almazari, Bilyana Azzam and Hanadi Abu Assab

Department of Clinical Pharmacy, Faculty of Pharmacy, Zarqa University, Zarqa 13132, Jordan; halhamad@zu.edu.jo (H.A.); ialmazari@zu.edu.jo (I.A.); bolbol.alazzam16@yahoo.com (B.A.); abuassabhanadi@gmail.com (H.A.A.)

* Correspondence: mabuassab@zu.edu.jo; Tel.: +962-795-902-490

Abstract: The medication review process (MRP) is an extended, vital role of community pharmacists in improving health outcomes of medication use, yet it is neither systematically nor comprehensively provided bycommunity pharmacies in Jordan. This study aimed to identify the potential barriers hinderingMRP implementation bycommunity pharmacists in Jordan. A total of 550 community pharmacists electronically received a previously constructed and validated Arabic questionnaire explicitly developed to assess the current medication review practices and factors hindering the MRP, of whom 417 answered the questionnaire, giving a response rate of 75.8%. Among the investigated six categories' seventeen barriers tothe implementation of the MRP, the highest rating was found for remuneration barriers (55.8%), followed by barriers related to regulations and patients, which scored 52.3% and 48.8%, respectively. Resource-related barriers were recognizedby 44.6% of participants, while qualifications and barriers related to physicians scored 42.9% and 41.8%, respectively. Although community pharmacists in Jordan are eager to extend their roles from traditional to more patient-centered ones, they encounter various barriers hinderingsuch development. Regulation adjustments accompanied by cost-effective remuneration and proper training are strong facilitators for community pharmacists to initiate the medication review service; make available the needed resources; and invest efforts, time, and money to operate it.

Keywords: medication review process; medication review service; pharmaceutical care; healthcare; barriers; community pharmacist; Jordan

Citation: Abu Assab, M.; Alhamad, H.; Almazari, I.; Azzam, B.; Abu Assab, H. Barriers to Medication Review Process Implementation—Cross-Sectional Study among Community Pharmacists in Jordan. *Healthcare* **2022**, *10*, 651. https://doi.org/10.3390/healthcare10040651

Academic Editor: Georges Adunlin

Received: 27 February 2022
Accepted: 25 March 2022
Published: 31 March 2022

1. Introduction

Recently, there has been an urgent need to broaden community pharmacists' roles in primary public health issues [1]. As a result, the range of services provided by community pharmacists has undergone rapid expansion, from traditional supply functions to more patient-focused services [2]. Community pharmacies comprise ideal sites for believable counseling that appeal to a large population segment. Furthermore, community pharmacists gain a unique understanding of the therapeutic management of the health needs of communities, operate underextended opening hours, and serve through daily interactions with patients, providing health education, immunization programs, disease awareness, and prevention initiatives [3]. The patient-centered roles of community pharmacists emphasize the achievement of optimal treatment results for the patient and the prevention ofhealth problems that patients may encounter because of the incorrect use of medicines [4]. The medication review process (MRP) is one of the crucial pharmaceutical care (PC) services that community pharmacists can provide, through which they perform a thorough review, evaluation, and discussion of patients' medications to obtain the best treatment plan and to prevent any medication-related health problems [5,6].

The MRP is defined as a systematic and structured critical evaluation of a patient's medicationto reach a treatment agreement, optimize medicationuse, minimize medication-related problems, improve health outcomes, and reduce waste [7,8]. According to the Pharmaceutical Care Network Europe (PCNE), a medication review (MR) is defined as a "structured evaluation of a patient's medicines with the aim to optimize medicines use and improving health outcomes" [9]. Therefore, the MRP is one of the most critical aspects of the PC process, through which a complete assessment of the patient's medications is carried out after determining the goals of the treatment and the patient's needs and taking into account all of the factors that affect the selection of the appropriate treatment plan for the disease condition, thus developing a treatment plan that ensures the right medicines with the right doses are provided to the right patient [10].

Studies addressed the MRP's positive outcomes on patients' life, particularly the elderly, who receive more than one drug for a long time. That is, the ultimate goal of the MRP is to obtain the best possible treatment plan, improve the patient's quality of life, reduce treatment costs, increase commitment to taking medication, and reduce potential medication-related side effects [10–21]. Therefore, the basis forconducting the process depends mainly on engaging indialogue with the patient to obtain all of the necessary information that mainly affects the treatment plan and the extent of the patient's commitment to taking the medications included in the treatment plan completely and appropriately, thus ensuringthat the correct patient receives the correct medication at the correct dose [22].

A couple of MRP-related local studies were conducted; the findings showed that the service had a positive impact on patients' health, that many problems related to the use of drugs were prevented from occurring when the MRP wasapplied, and that there wasacceptance and satisfaction from the patients about pharmacists performing the process due to the positive results on the patients' health [23,24].

Although the MRP is widely adopted and studied globally [13,25], it is seldom provided bycommunity pharmacies in Jordan [23,24]. There is a lack of studies that address the potential barriers that hinderthe adoption of such a service bycommunity pharmacies.

This study aimed to identify the potential barriers hinderingMRP implementation bycommunity pharmacists in Jordan, and it is expected to be the first in Jordan to do so. The outcomes of this study are valuable to supplement the decisionmakers (such as the Jordan Pharmacists Association (JPA)) with the key barriers and obstacles hinderingthe comprehensive implementation of the medication review service (MRS) by community pharmacists, thus enabling them to articulate plans and policies to bridge the gap between the current roles performed by community pharmacists and the needed future broader patient-centered roles.

2. Materials and Methods

Study design and settings: This was an observational, cross-sectional studyusing a pre-tested, validated questionnaire distributed to a sample of community pharmacies in Jordan. Data were collected over three months (from April to June 2021). Figure S1 depicts a flowchart of the whole study process.

Study instrument: The study questionnaire was developed based on previous studies, a literature review [11,13,14,22–24], and research objectives. It was designed to be in Arabic to support participants' responses, as Arabic is the official and mother-tongue language in Jordan. Six experts and five clinical pharmacists were individually approached to participate in the questionnaire validation process. Furthermore, a pilot study was performed to ensure that the questions were clear, understandable, and reflected the study's objectives. Thirty community pharmacies were selected randomly, and the questionnaire with the study objectives was sent to them electronically, inviting them to participate. The pilot questionnaire electronic responses were collected over three weeks and tested for consistency and reliability before initiating the formal data collection process. Then, the updated, refined questionnaire was distributed electronically through social media (community pharmacies' Whatsapp and Facebook groups), where pharmacists were invited to participate in the study questionnaire.

Sample size calculation and sampling strategy: According to JPA, there are currently around 3700 community pharmacies, with approximately 7200 community pharmacists. At a 95% confidence level and a 5% margin of error (significance $\alpha = 0.05$) with a 50% response distribution, the minimum sample size was calculated to be 365 [26]. The questionnaire was distributed to a sample of 550 community pharmacies.

Inclusion and exclusion criteria: The study participants were pharmacists working in community pharmacies in Jordan. All other pharmacy staff members and pharmacists working in settings other than community pharmacies were excluded.

Questionnaire measures: The electronic questionnaire contained three parts: the first was designed to obtain the socio-demographic characteristics of respondents, the second was dedicated to investigating the MRP implementation practices and behaviors performed by community pharmacists, and the third part was dedicated to identifying the barriers to MRP implementation that community pharmacists in Jordan recognize.

Data analysis: The Statistical Package for Social Science (SPSS) software, version 23, was used to analyze the data generated from the study. The participants' demographics arepresented using descriptive statistics (frequency/percentage). For the assessment of MRP practices and behavior questionnaire items (part two; 8 items), the Likert's agreement five-point response scale (strongly disagree to strongly agree) was used. The Likert five-point response scale of frequency (never to always) was used to assess the barriers related to MRP implementation that community pharmacists in Jordan recognize(part three; 17 items). Descriptive statistics (frequency/percentage) were utilized to present responses on each scale, and missing responses were excluded from the calculation ofresponse percentages to the survey items.

3. Results

A total of 550 community pharmacies from 12 governorates were approached to participate in the study, of which 417 answered the questionnaire, giving a response rate of 75.8%.

3.1. The Socio-Demographic Characteristics of the Participants

An overview of the socio-demographic characteristics of the participants is presented in Table 1. The majority of participants were female ($n = 321$, 77.0%), hadan age ranging from 25 to less than 35 years ($n = 212$, 50.8%), had a BSc degree in pharmacy ($n = 335$, 80.3%), worked in independent pharmacies ($n = 315$, 75.5%), were from the northern governorates ($n = 234$, 56.1%), and had 3 years or less of working experience in community pharmacies ($n = 240$, 57.6%), and most of them were staff pharmacists ($n = 317$, 76.0%).

Table 1. Socio-demographic characteristics of the participants (N = 417).

Characteristic		N	%
Gender	Female	321	77.0
	Male	92	22.0
	Missing data	4	1.0
Age	25 to less than 35 years	212	50.8
	35 to less than 45 years	45	10.8
	More than 45 years	34	8.2
	Less than 25 years	123	29.5
	Missing data	3	0.7

Table 1. *Cont.*

Characteristic		N	%
Qualification	Bachelor (Doctor of Pharmacy)	27	6.5
	Bachelor (pharmacy)	335	80.3
	Ph.D.	2	0.5
	Master's degree	40	9.6
	Missing data	13	3.1
The governorate in which the pharmacy is located	Central governorates	163	39.1
	Southern governorates	17	4.1
	Northern governorates	234	56.1
	Missing data	3	0.7
Pharmacy Ownership	Chain pharmacy	89	21.4
	Independent pharmacy	315	75.5
	Missing data	13	3.1
Job Title	Pharmacist owner	20	4.8
	Owner and responsible pharmacist	50	12.0
	Employee pharmacist	317	76.0
	Other	18	4.2
	Missing data	13	3.0
Practical experience in community pharmacies	More than 10 years	51	12.2
	3-6 years	69	16.5
	6-10 years	51	12.2
	Less than 3 years	240	57.6
	Missing data	6	1.5

3.2. *Reliability of Questionnaire*

Questionnaire consistency and reliability were measured using Cronbach's α test, where the overall internal consistency was excellent (Cronbach's $\alpha = 0.920$), with Cronbach's α measures ranging from 0.901 to 0.950.

3.3. *MRP Implementation Practices and Behaviors Performed by Community Pharmacists in Jordan*

Table 2 shows the MRP practices and behaviors performed by community pharmacists in Jordan. The assessment revealed that 71.7% of them perform practices and behaviors related to the MRP, as 49.4% of them collect relevant data from patients or their caregivers. This is followed by the assessment of whether the prescribed medication is appropriate for the patient's condition and whether the prescribed medications may cause health problems depending on the patient's condition, at 48.0% and 45.8%, respectively. A total of41.7% of respondents stated that they are constantly improving their skills to conduct specialized MR. The assessment of whether the patient is satisfied with continuing the treatment and whether the patient still needs all of his/her medication was reported by 40.5% and 38.6% of respondents, respectively. Developing a plan that includes a follow-up with treating physicians and documenting the files of patients who underwent the MRP were performed by 36.7% and 33.3% of respondents, respectively.

Table 2. Medication review process (MRP) practices and behaviors performed by community pharmacists in Jordan (N = 417).

Rank	Practice/Behavior	N	%
1	We collect relevant information from patients or their caregivers.	206	49.4
2	We assess whether the prescribed medication is appropriate for the patient's condition.	200	48.0
3	We assess whether the prescribed medications may cause health problems depending on the patient's condition.	191	45.8
4	We are constantly improving our skills to conduct specialized medication reviews.	174	41.7
5	We assess whether the patient is satisfied with continuing the treatment.	169	40.5
6	We assess whether the patient still needs all of his/her medications.	161	38.6
7	We develop a plan that includes follow-up with the patient's treating physician.	153	36.7
8	We have documentation (manual or electronic records) of patients' profiles to conducting the medication review process.	139	33.3

3.4. Barriers to MRP Implementation

Table 3 shows the reactions of Jordanian community pharmacists to 17 barriers to implementing the MRP, grouped into six categories: patient-related, physician-related, and resource-related barriers, in addition to regulation-related, qualification-related, and remuneration-related barriers. The highest rating was found for remuneration barriers (55.8%), followed by barriers related to regulations and patients, which scored 52.3% and 48.8%, respectively. Resource-related barriers were recognized by 44.6% of participants, while qualifications and barriers related to physicians scored 42.9% and 41.8%, respectively.

Table 3. Barriers to MRP implementation bycommunity pharmacists in Jordan (N = 417).

Rank	Barrier Category (%)	Barrier Items	N	%
1	Remuneration related (55.8%)	Insurers are ready to cover a fee for the pharmacist to perform the medication review process for their insured patients.	86	20.6
		Patients are willing to pay the pharmacist for the medication review process.	87	20.9
		The pharmacy provides a financial incentive for pharmacists who conduct medication re-views	130	31.2
2	Regulation related (52.3%)	There is an approved reference and specific steps for the pharmacist to carry out the medica-tion review process.	95	22.8
3	Patient related (48.8%)	Patients accept the medication review process by the pharmacist.	82	19.7
		The patients provide the pharmacist with the information needed to perform the medication review process.	128	30.7
4	Resource related (44.6%)	We can provide enough time to do the medication review process.	119	28.5
		Doing a medication review requires the availability of specialized databases.	203	48.7
		Implementing the medication review process requires the appointment of a pharmacist dedi-cated to this purpose.	174	41.7
		The medication review process requires a designated place in the pharmacy.	166	39.8
		The pharmacy management supports the medication review process.	156	37.4
		Performing medication reviews is a waste of a pharmacist's time.	79	18.9
5	Qualification related (42.9%)	Pharmacists have sufficient training and practical applications to conduct the medication re-view process.	98	23.5
		The medication review process is taught during the undergraduate level.	126	30.2
		Qualified and trained pharmacists are available to carry out the medication review process.	140	33.6

Table 3. *Cont.*

Rank	Barrier Category (%)	Barrier Items	N	%
6	Physician related (41.8%)	The treating physician accepts the results and outcomes of the medication review process.	95	22.8
		The success of the medication review process requires good relationships with the treating physicians.	204	48.9

4. Discussion

Although the MRP is widely adopted and studied globally, it is neither systematically nor comprehensively provided by community pharmacies in Jordan. Moreover, there is a lack of studies that address the potential barriers that hinder the adoption of such a service by community pharmacies.

Data from a Jordanian study showed that the main barriers recognized to hinder the implementation of PC were pharmacists' lack of pharmaceutical training (44.9%), lack of acceptability by physicians (43.4%), lack of supporting laws (42.0%), pharmacists' lack of therapeutic knowledge and clinical problem-solving skills (39.4%), and pharmacists' lack of communication skills (38.2%) [27]. Six categories of barriers were identified throughout this research.

The majority of the community pharmacists believed that neither insurance nor patients were willing to pay for the MRS. Studies showed that conducting services such as MR would necessitate greater resources, such as additional staff, and, hence, necessitate an appropriate remuneration scheme. They also showed that adequate remuneration is an important facilitator for providing this type of service. Time and resource burdens are not problematic if the remuneration is adequate [11,14]. On the national level, given the current economic constraints, community pharmacists believed that paying for this service would be problematic and perhaps impede the adoption of such a service. Thus, healthcare benefits, notably safety, effectiveness, and cost management, must still be shown to policymakers to secure funding from health insurance companies, the government, and patients. Although adequate remuneration is necessary to allow initial investments, it is not the only facilitator of the provision of this kind of service and is generally not sufficient alone to put a new service into action in community pharmacies' practice [11,14].

Community pharmacies' legal conduct in Jordan is regulated through three central legislations, namely, the General Health Act, the Medication and Pharmacy Act, and the Jordan Pharmacists Association (JPA) Act. The provision of health and PC services bycommunity pharmacies, other than the preparation and dispensing of medications with related counseling to patients, is neither stated nor defined in these legislations; hence, community pharmacists must consider the regulation barriers to providing MR and any service. This study shows that only 22.7% of respondents believe that there is an approved reference for the service administration. In 2019, after a focused extensive effort by JPA, qualified community pharmacists were legally allowed to administer flu vaccination. JPA also exerts extra efforts in a similar direction to transform community pharmacists' roles into more extended patient-centered ones. Such leaps are vital in facilitating PC services, including MR and medication therapy management (MTM).

The patient is the merit of the MRP, and his/her inclusion is the first step of its implementation. Thus, patient-related obstacles are at the heart of the process. The findings of this study show that less than one-quarter of the community pharmacists stated that patients accepted the pharmacist's proposal to perform the MRP and that only 30.7% of them believed that patients provided them with enough information needed to perform the process. A study showed that patients' refusal of the pharmacists' proposal to be involved in the MRP could be attributed to several factors, including whether they think they do not need this service or whether they think that it is not the role of pharmacists. Some do not come to the pharmacy by themselves [11]. However, implementation of the MRP will be more straightforward if patients already have a good relationship with the pharmacist. Additional support, such as a broad media plan/program, to increase their awareness and perceptions toward the MRS and to highlight the benefits of this service on patients' outcomes, particularly those with chronic disease and polypharmacy patients, will be the necessary beneficial facilitator. Concerning access to patient information, a study concluded that the lack of access to patient health information is an essential obstacle to MTM interventions. Access to electronic health records could help in this area [28]. However, this type of research is absent in Jordan, and further research is essential to determine the benefit of electronic health record access in community pharmacies. It will be a crucial future leap in community pharmacy-based patient-centered services. On a related front, almost 33% of community pharmacists in this study stated that they have documentation (manual or electronic records) of patients' profiles to conduct the MRP. We can currently assume that those community pharmacists individually use their initiatives to develop and deliver services to their patients. In this instance, our focus throughout this study was primarily directed to identify the potential barriers hindering MRP implementation by community pharmacists in Jordan. Future research is needed by those who perform medication reviews to investigate their level of MRS implementation.

The majority of the community pharmacists who participated seemed unable to invest time and resources in developing new services. Concerning time, 71.5% of community pharmacists stated that they lack the time for the MRP; these findings are in line with studies on the MRP [11,14]. While the "lack of time" obstacle has frequently been noted in pharmacy practice research, this obstacle is caused by a lack of staff, directly tied to a lack of remuneration for this type of service. It is exacerbated by the pharmacy's severe workload and administrative burden [29–34]. Therefore, time and resource constraints are not problematic if adequate remuneration is embraced [11,14]. Furthermore, pharmacists need to learn to delegate tasks better within their teams to make time in their already busy schedules. Efficient delegation requires good team communication within the pharmacy and special training for staff [11].

Our study shows that 48.7%, 41.7%, and 39.8% of pharmacists believe that the MRP needs a particular database, an appointment arrangement, and a dedicated place, respectively. Even though MRS in daily practice requires appropriate workflow management, such as physical space dedicated to conducting patient interviews and particular platforms, a dearth of research assesses the significance of this issue. A study investigated the barriers related to health information exchange that limit the ability to access and share accurate, complete, and timely medication data across the care spectrum and suggested several strategies to promote reliable data sharing across many systems with integrated data sharing infrastructures (e.g., plans, electronic health records, pharmacy systems, retail systems, and personal applications). Emerging technologies, such as digital therapies, pharmacogenomics, precision medicine, and artificial intelligence-driven services, will require such infrastructures. In addition, the rising body of evidence suggests that embracing a paradigm change in data ownership and management, in which individuals play an increasingly central role in accessing, owning, and re-sharing their data across their lives, can lead to revolutionary progress [35].

Commitment, support, and engagement from community pharmacies' owners and top management are crucial for the successful implementation of any service. Unfortunately, only 37.4% of the study respondents reported that they gained the owners/pharmacy managers' support for the MRP. Fortunately, only 18.9% of the participants believed that the MRP was a waste of time. This issue implies that community pharmacists in Jordan address the importance of the MRP and that most of them are eager to carry it out formally in their pharmacies.

In alignment with other studies [11,23,36], this study's findings reveal that a lack of adequate training related to the MRP isa significant barrier, as only 23.5% of participating community pharmacists had sufficient training and practical application on how to conduct the service. In addition, only 30.2% of respondents stated that the MRP was taught at the undergraduate level, and 33.6% believed that there are no qualified ortrained pharmacists to carry out this process. One study from Jordan reported that the provision of PC is limited and that the lack of PC training is a significant barrier for PC implementation [36]. Training appears to be an essential facilitator of the practice change process in community pharmacies [37]. Jordanian community pharmacists are seriously concerned about training and clinical skills, as are pharmacists in many other countries regarding patient-centered care and health promotion [27]. The training goals for the implementation of the MRP must include essential high-level pharmacotherapy (tailored to primary care practice), pharmacoeconomics, and services, as well as management skills and specific medicine review abilities (for example, selecting patients and who has priority; conducting data analysis to identify eligible patients; conducting patient interviews; and writing reports). Computer skills are also required (data management and outcome monitoring) [38,39]. Policymakers should keep training in mind when planning strategies to adopt modern programs or services, and academics should incorporate these features into pharmacist training. Changes in undergraduate pharmacy curricula are required to guarantee that students learn more about patient-focused issues and the relevant parts of information management and technology, behavioral sciences, communication, and health problem solving. Doing so will ensure that the students gain the necessary information and skills for patient care practice. It is critical to introduce postgraduate programs that place a greater emphasis on patient-centered teaching and training. Wherever possible, pharmacy schools should be administratively positioned so that the combined training of health professionals is possible. Pharmacy owners should also be aware of the need to involve their entire workforce in the implementation process, even if the service is seemingly supplied solely by the pharmacist, and should engage staff members in the planning and goal-setting procedures.

Establishing a good relationship with the treating physician is essential for the success of the MRP, as this study reveals that only 22.7% of community pharmacists believe that the patients' physician will accept the results and outcomes of the MRP and that 48.9% of them believe that a good relationship is required for successful implementation of the service. Despite the many benefits of establishing and maintaining positive relationships between community pharmacists and physicians, doing so is not always straightforward. The need for collaborative practice agreements has been documented in the pharmacy literature worldwide [40–43]. Another critical study about physicians' attitudes toward pharmacist-provided MTM treatments emphasized the importance of direct joint pharmacist–physician coordination of care [44]. However, a study showed that physicians in Jordan accept the pharmacist's traditional role. They are, however, apprehensive of the adoption of additional clinical responsibilities [45]. According to a study, the development of inter-professional workshops in collaboration with various healthcare associations might be examined to allow pharmacists and physicians the opportunity to meet face to face and discuss shared objectives [46]. In addition, changes to reimbursement models and infrastructures, such as province-wide drug information systems and electronic health records, may be needed to realize the full benefit of collaborative practice between pharmacists and physicians to achieve optimal quality and outcomes of patient care [47]. Thus, we need to develop strategies and interventions to encourage collaboration with a more profound knowledge of the physician's connection. The most vital strategies to implement are to encourage positive attitudes and the perception of helpfulness, and for health administrators and professionals to take advantage of new changes enforced by the health system as an opportunity to initiate collaboration, as well as promoting face-to-face relationship development to overcome prejudices, enable teamwork initiation and development, and designate coordinators responsibilities. Future studies are required to assess the efficacy of these tactics, as well as the further assessment of physicians' perceptions toward the MRP in Jordan.

Although the findings of our study in Jordan are almost comparable to those of other studies conducted in other countries worldwide, we needed to conduct this study to determine where we are currently, what our ground base is regarding the barriers to MRP implementation, and where to start building the capacity for the service in Jordan.

Comprehensively, a multi-stakeholder engagement approach that involves pharmacy colleges, professional associations (pharmacists and physicians), health policymakers, and health insurance is essential for the development and practice implementation of the MRS.

4.1. Study Strengths and Limitations

This study is expected to be the first or among the few that addressed the potential barriers that hinder the adoption of MRS by community pharmacies in Jordan. Thus, this study's outcomes are valuable foundations to supplement the decisionmakers, such as JPA, with the key barriers and obstacles hindering the comprehensive implementation of the service by community pharmacists, consequently enabling them to articulate plans and policies to bridge the gap between the current roles performed by community pharmacists and the needed future broader patient-centered roles.

This research was conducted during the ongoing COVID-19 pandemic, explaining the use of an electronically distributed questionnaire as a data collection tool, giving rise to a sort of response bias toward youth community pharmacists with higher interaction; follow-up; and familiarity with electronic, digital, and social media platforms compared to older counterparts.

For future research, we suggest, if possible, establishing a list of all licensed community pharmacies in Jordan with their geographic distribution and using both electronically and personally distributed surveys to ensure the representation of all community pharmacists' age groups and governorates where pharmacies are located.

4.2. Implications for Future Research

The investigation of the level of MRS implementation by community pharmacists who perform medication reviews and the proposal of a feasible business model for community pharmacy-based MRSs are areas of future research interest to whoever is concerned with optimizing health and economic outcomes of medications and other therapies for the population of Jordan.

5. Conclusions

Our study identified six categories of barriers that currently hinder MRP implementation by community pharmacists in Jordan. The findings from this study pave the way for health policymakers and decisionmakers, such as JPA and the Ministry of Health, to develop plans and policies to effectively and efficiently take advantage of community pharmacies' capacity to serve patients and the healthcare system as a whole, explicitly removing the constraints that hinder community pharmacists' adoption and execution of more prominent patient-centered roles. Regulation adjustments to allow community pharmacists to exert the MRP, accompanied by a cost-effective remuneration scheme and proper training, are solid motivators for community pharmacies to initiate the service; make needed resources available; and invest efforts, time, and money to operate it.

Supplementary Materials: The following supporting information can be downloaded at: https://www.mdpi.com/article/10.3390/healthcare10040651/s1. Figure S1: Flowchart of the whole study process.

Author Contributions: Conceptualization, M.A.A. and B.A.; data curation, M.A.A., H.A., B.A. and H.A.A.; formal analysis, M.A.A., H.A., B.A. and H.A.A.; funding acquisition, M.A.A.; investigation, H.A., I.A., B.A. and H.A.A.; methodology, M.A.A., H.A., I.A., B.A. and H.A.A.; project administration, M.A.A.; resources, M.A.A. and I.A.; software, I.A.; supervision, H.A. and I.A.; validation, H.A. and H.A.A.; visualization, I.A.; writing—original draft, M.A.A., H.A., I.A., B.A. and H.A.A.; writing—review and editing, M.A.A., H.A., I.A., B.A. and H.A.A. All authors have read and agreed to the published version of the manuscript.

Funding: This research received no external funding.

Institutional Review Board Statement: This study was conducted according to the guidelines of the Declaration of Helsinki and approved by the Clinical Pharmacy Department and the Scientific Research Committee/Faculty of Pharmacy/Zarqa University (approval decision number 24/2021/2022 date 22 December 2021).

Informed Consent Statement: Informed consent was obtained from all subjects involved in the study.

Data Availability Statement: The data presented in this study are available on request from the corresponding author.

Conflicts of Interest: The authors declare no conflict of interest.

References

1. O'Loughlin, J.; Masson, P.; Déry, V.; Fagnan, D. The Role of Community Pharmacists in Health Education and Disease Prevention: A Survey of Their Interests and Needs in Relation to Cardiovascular Disease. *Prev. Med.* **1999**, *28*, 324–331. [CrossRef] [PubMed]
2. Thomson, K.; Hillier-Brown, F.; Walton, N.; Bilaj, M.; Bambra, C.; Todd, A. The Effects of Community Pharmacy-Delivered Public Health Interventions on Population Health and Health Inequalities: A Review of Reviews. *Prev. Med.* **2019**, *124*, 98–109. [CrossRef] [PubMed]
3. Laliberté, M.-C.; Perreault, S.; Damestoy, N.; Lalonde, L. Ideal and Actual Involvement of Community Pharmacists in Health Promotion and Prevention: A Cross-Sectional Study in Quebec, Canada. *BMC Public Health* **2012**, *12*, 192. [CrossRef] [PubMed]
4. Almarsdóttir, A.B.; Granas, A.G.; Blondal, A.B. Clinical and Social Perspectives on Pharmacy Services. In *Clinical Pharmacy Education, Practice and Research*; Elsevier: Amsterdam, The Netherlands, 2019; pp. 31–40.
5. Khera, S.; Abbasi, M.; Dabravolskaj, J.; Sadowski, C.A.; Yua, H.; Chevalier, B. Appropriateness of Medications in Older Adults Living with Frailty: Impact of a Pharmacist-Led Structured Medication Review Process in Primary Care. *J. Prim. Care Community Health* **2019**, *10*, 2150132719890227. [CrossRef]
6. Aronson, J.K. Medication Errors: What They Are, How They Happen, and How to Avoid Them. *QJM* **2009**, *102*, 513–521. [CrossRef] [PubMed]
7. Geurts, M.M.E.; Talsma, J.; Brouwers, J.R.B.J.; de Gier, J.J. Medication Review and Reconciliation with Cooperation between Pharmacist and General Practitioner and the Benefit for the Patient: A Systematic Review: Cooperation between Pharmacist and General Practitioner. *Br. J. Clin. Pharmacol.* **2012**, *74*, 16–33. [CrossRef] [PubMed]
8. Malet-Larrea, A.; Goyenechea, E.; García-Cárdenas, V.; Calvo, B.; Arteche, J.M.; Aranegui, P.; Zubeldia, J.J.; Gastelurrutia, M.A.; Martínez-Martínez, F.; Benrimoj, S.I. The Impact of a Medication Review with Follow-up Service on Hospital Admissions in Aged Polypharmacy Patients: Impact of the Medication Review with Follow-up on Hospital Admissions. *Br. J. Clin. Pharmacol.* **2016**, *82*, 831–838. [CrossRef] [PubMed]
9. Griese-Mammen, N.; Hersberger, K.E.; Messerli, M.; Leikola, S.; Horvat, N.; van Mil, J.W.F.; Kos, M. PCNE Definition of Medication Review: Reaching Agreement. *Int. J. Clin. Pharm.* **2018**, *40*, 1199–1208. [CrossRef]
10. Blenkinsopp, A.; Bond, C.; Raynor, D.K. Medication Reviews: Medication Reviews. *Br. J. Clin. Pharmacol.* **2012**, *74*, 573–580. [CrossRef]
11. Niquille, A.; Lattmann, C.; Bugnon, O. Medication Reviews Led by Community Pharmacists in Switzerland: A Qualitative Survey to Evaluate Barriers and Facilitators. *Pharm. Pract.* **2010**, *8*, 35–42. [CrossRef] [PubMed]
12. Berenguer, B.; La Casa, C.; de la Matta, M.J.; Martín-Calero, M.J. Pharmaceutical Care: Past, Present and Future. *Curr. Pharm. Des.* **2004**, *10*, 3931–3946. [CrossRef] [PubMed]
13. Brandt, J.; Lê, M.-L.; Jantscher, S.; Bricelj, A.; Louizos, C.; Ng, S.; Sibley, K. Medication Review Service Implementation in Com-Munity Pharmacy Settings: Scoping Review with Focus on Implementation Studies. *Res. Social Adm. Pharm.* **2020**, *16*, 875–885. [CrossRef] [PubMed]
14. Lelubre, M.; Wuyts, J.; Maesschalck, J.; Duquet, N.; Foubert, K.; Hutsebaut, C.; Moullin, J.; De Wulf, I.; Boussery, K.; Foulon, V.; et al. Implementation Study of an Intermediate Medication Review in Belgian Community Pharmacies. *Res. Soc. Adm. Pharm.* **2019**, *15*, 710–723. [CrossRef]
15. Palleria, C.; Di Paolo, A.; Giofrè, C.; Caglioti, C.; Leuzzi, G.; Siniscalchi, A.; De Sarro, G.; Gallelli, L. Pharmacokinetic Drug-Drug Interaction and Their Implication in Clinical Management. *J. Res. Med. Sci.* **2013**, *18*, 601–610.
16. Verdoorn, S.; Kwint, H.-F.; Blom, J.W.; Gussekloo, J.; Bouvy, M.L. Effects of a Clinical Medication Review Focused on Personal Goals, Quality of Life, and Health Problems in Older Persons with Polypharmacy: A Randomised Controlled Trial (DREA-MeR-Study). *PLoS Med.* **2019**, *16*, 114. [CrossRef] [PubMed]
17. Awad, A.; Alhadab, A.; Albassam, A. Medication-Related Burden and Medication Adherence among Geriatric Patients in Kuwait: A Cross-Sectional Study. *Front. Pharmacol.* **2020**, *11*, 1296. [CrossRef] [PubMed]
18. Chau, S.H.; Jansen, A.P.D.; van de Ven, P.M.; Hoogland, P.; Elders, P.J.M.; Hugtenburg, J.G. Clinical Medication Reviews in Elderly Patients with Polypharmacy: A Cross-Sectional Study on Drug-Related Problems in the Netherlands. *Int. J. Clin. Pharm.* **2016**, *38*, 46–53. [CrossRef] [PubMed]
19. Schindler, E.; Hohmann, C.; Culmsee, C. Medication Review by Community Pharmacists for Type 2 Diabetes Patients in Rou-Tine Care: Results of the DIATHEM-Study. *Front. Pharmacol.* **2020**, *14*, 1176. [CrossRef]
20. Smith, W. Adverse Drug Reactions—Allergy? Side-Effect? Intolerance? *Aust. Fam. Physician* **2013**, *42*, 12–16. [PubMed]

21. Farooqui, R.; Hoor, T.; Karim, N.; Muneer, M. Potential Drug-Drug Interactions among Patients Prescriptions Collected from Medicine Out-Patient Setting. *Pak. J. Med. Sci. Q.* **2018**, *34*, 144–148. [CrossRef] [PubMed]
22. Brandt, M.; Hallas, J.; Graabæk, T.; Pottegård, A. Description of a Practice Model for Pharmacist Medication Review in a General Practice Setting. *Pharm. Pract.* **2014**, *12*, 420. [CrossRef] [PubMed]
23. Basheti, I.A.; Tadros, O.K.I.; Aburuz, S. Value of a Community-Based Medication Management Review Service in Jordan: A Prospective Randomized Controlled Study. *Pharmacotherapy* **2016**, *36*, 1075–1086. [CrossRef]
24. Basheti, I.A.; Tadros, O.K.I.; Alnajjar, M.S.; Aburuz, S. Assessing Patient Satisfaction with the Medication Management Review Service Delivered in Jordan. *J. Pharm. Health Serv. Res.* **2019**, *10*, 49–55. [CrossRef]
25. Imfeld-Isenegger, T.L.; Soares, I.B.; Makovec, U.N.; Horvat, N.; Kos, M.; van Mil, F.; Costa, F.A.; Hersberger, K.E. Communitypharmacist-led medication review procedures across Europe: Characterization, implementation and remuneration. *Res. Soc. Adm. Pharm.* **2020**, *16*, 1057–1066. [CrossRef] [PubMed]
26. Raosoft, Inc. Sample Size Calculator. Available online: http://www.raosoft.com/samplesize.html (accessed on 26 February 2022).
27. Elayeh, E.; Akour, A.; Almadaeen, S.; AlQhewii, T.; Basheti, I.A. Practice of Pharmaceutical Care in Community Pharmacies in Jordan. *Trop. J. Pharm. Res.* **2017**, *16*, 463. [CrossRef]
28. Roberts, M.F.; Reeves, K.; Divine, H. Community Pharmacists' Lack of Access to Health Records and Its Impact on Targeted MTM Interventions. *J. Am. Pharm. Assoc.* **2019**, *59*, S81–S84. [CrossRef] [PubMed]
29. Mahmoud, A. Barriers for Implementation of Pharmaceutical Care Practice in Community Pharmacies in Sudan. *Khartoum Med. J.* **2014**, *7*, 921–931.
30. Hajj, M.S.; Al-Saeed, H.S.; Khaja, M. Qatar Pharmacists' Understanding, Attitudes, Practice and Perceived Barriers Related to Providing Pharmaceutical Care. *Int. J. Clin. Pharm.* **2016**, *38*, 330–343. [CrossRef] [PubMed]
31. Blake, K.B.; Madhavan, S.S.; Scott, V.G.; Meredith Elswick, B.L. Medication Therapy Management Services in West Virginia: Pharmacists' Perceptions of Educational and Training Needs. *Res. Soc. Adm. Pharm.* **2009**, *5*, 182–188. [CrossRef] [PubMed]
32. Hohmeier, K.C.; Wheeler, J.; Heintz, K.; Gatwood, J. Community Pharmacist Workflow and Medication Therapy Management Delegation. An Assessment of Preferences and Barriers. *J. Am. Pharm. Assoc.* **2020**, *60*, e215–e223. [CrossRef] [PubMed]
33. Law, A.V.; Okamoto, M.P.; Brock, K. Ready, Willing, and Able to Provide MTM Services? A Survey of Community Pharmacists in the USA. *Res. Soc. Adm. Pharm.* **2009**, *5*, 376–381. [CrossRef] [PubMed]
34. Sherman, J.J. Medication Therapy Management Challenges in Patients with Diabetes: A Systematic Review. *US Pharm.* **2015**, *10*, 16.
35. Thornewill, J.; Antimisiaris, D.; Ezekekwu, E.; Esterhay, R. Transformational Strategies for Optimizing Use of Medications and Related Therapies through Us Pharmacists and Pharmacies: Findings from a National Study. *J. Am. Pharm. Assoc.* **2021**, *62*, 450–460. [CrossRef]
36. Aburuz, S.; Al-Ghazawi, M.; Snyder, A. Pharmaceutical Care in a Community-Based Practice Setting in Jordan: Where Are We Now with Our Attitudes and Perceived Barriers? Pharmaceutical Care in Jordan. *Int. J. Pharm. Pract.* **2012**, *20*, 71–79. [CrossRef] [PubMed]
37. Roberts, A.S.; Benrimoj, S.I.; Chen, T.F.; Williams, K.A.; Aslani, P. Practice Change in Community Pharmacy: Quantification of Facilitators. *Ann. Pharmacother.* **2008**, *42*, 861–868. [CrossRef] [PubMed]
38. Hassali, M.; Palaian, S.; Shafie, A.; Ibrahim, M. Perceptions and Barriers towards Provision of Health Promotion Activities among Community Pharmacists in the State of Penang. *J. Clin. Diagn. Res.* **2009**, *3*, 1562–1568.
39. Dunlop, J.A.; Shaw, J.P. Community Pharmacists' Perspectives on Pharmaceutical Care Implementation in New Zealand. *Pharm. World Sci.* **2002**, *24*, 224–230. [CrossRef] [PubMed]
40. Bacci, J.L.; Coley, K.C.; McGrath, K.; Abraham, O.; Adams, A.J.; McGivney, M.S. Strategies to Facilitate the Implementation of Collaborative Practice Agreements in Chain Community Pharmacies. *J. Am. Pharm. Assoc.* **2016**, *56*, 257–265.e2. [CrossRef] [PubMed]
41. Brock, K.A.; Doucette, W.R. Collaborative Working Relationships between Pharmacists and Physicians: An Exploratory Study. *J. Am. Pharm. Assoc.* **2004**, *44*, 358–365. [CrossRef] [PubMed]
42. Chui, M.A.; Stone, J.A.; Odukoya, O.K.; Maxwell, L. Facilitating Collaboration between Pharmacists and Physicians Using an Iterative Interview Process. *J. Am. Pharm. Assoc.* **2014**, *54*, 35–41. [CrossRef]
43. Foundation, A.P.A.; Benjamin, M. Association, Consortium Recommendations for Advancing Pharmacists' Patient Care Services and Collaborative Practice Agreements. *J. Am. Pharm. Assoc.* **2013**, *53*, e132–e141.
44. Mcgrath, S.H.; Snyder, M.E.; Dueñas, G.G.; Pringle, J.L.; Smith, R.B.; Mcgivney, M.S. Physician Perceptions of Pharmac-Ist-Provided Medication Therapy Management: Qualitative Analysis. *J. Am. Pharm. Assoc.* **2010**, *50*, 67–71. [CrossRef] [PubMed]
45. Tahaineh, L.M.; Wazaify, M.; Albsoul-Younes, A.; Khader, Y.; Zaidan, M. Perceptions, Experiences, and Expectations of Physi-Cians in Hospital Settings in Jordan Regarding the Role of the Pharmacist. *Res. Soc. Adm. Pharm.* **2009**, *5*, 63–70. [CrossRef]
46. Rubio-Valera, M.; Jové, A.M.; Hughes, C.M.; Guillen-Solà, M.; Rovira, M.; Fernández, A. Factors Affecting Collaboration between General Practitioners and Community Pharmacists: A Qualitative Study. *BMC Health Serv. Res.* **2012**, *12*, 188. [CrossRef] [PubMed]
47. Kelly, D.V.; Bishop, L.; Young, S.; Hawboldt, J.; Phillips, L.; Keough, T.M. Pharmacist and Physician Views on Collaborative Practice: Findings from the Community Pharmaceutical Care Project: Findings from the Community Pharmaceutical Care Project. *Can. Pharm. J.* **2013**, *146*, 218–226. [CrossRef] [PubMed]

healthcare

MDPI

Systematic Review

Practices and Perceptions of Community Pharmacists in the Management of Atopic Dermatitis: A Systematic Review and Thematic Synthesis

Abdi Berk Cayci [1,2,*], Adam Pattison Rathbone [1] and Laura Lindsey [1]

1 School of Pharmacy, Faculty of Medical Sciences, Newcastle University, Newcastle upon Tyne NE1 7RU, UK; adam.rathbone@ncl.ac.uk (A.P.R.); laura.lindsey@ncl.ac.uk (L.L.)

2 Faculty of Pharmacy, Hacettepe University, Ankara 06100, Türkiye

* Correspondence: a.b.cayci2@newcastle.ac.uk

Abstract: Understanding the contributions of community pharmacists as first-line health providers is important to the management of atopic dermatitis, though little is known about their contribution. A systematic review was carried out to examine practices and perceptions of the role of community pharmacists. A literature search was conducted in five different databases. Full-text primary research studies, which involved practices and perceptions of the role of community pharmacists in the management of atopic dermatitis, previously published in peer reviewed journals were used. Critical appraisal of included studies was performed using the Mixed Methods Appraisal Tool. Data were extracted and thematically synthesized to generate descriptive and analytical themes. The confidence of the findings of the included studies was assessed via either GRADE or CERQual. Twenty-three studies were included. Findings showed that community pharmacists lacked knowledge of the uses of topical corticosteroids. The recommendations of other treatments were limited. Pharmacists generally undertook dermatology training after graduation. Analytical themes indicated that the practices of community pharmacists were poor and misled patients. Inappropriate education in initial training was identified as a potential reason for their poor practices. This systematic review reveals a gap between patients' needs in practice and dermatological education provided to community pharmacists. Novel approaches regarding education and training should be explored to improve pharmacists' dermatological knowledge and skills.

Keywords: atopic dermatitis; community pharmacist; pharmacy practice; pharmacy education; systematic review

check for updates

Citation: Cayci, A.B.; Rathbone, A.P.; Lindsey, L. Practices and Perceptions of Community Pharmacists in the Management of Atopic Dermatitis: A Systematic Review and Thematic Synthesis. *Healthcare* **2023**, *11*, 2159. https://doi.org/10.3390/healthcare11152159

Academic Editor: Georges Adunlin

Received: 25 June 2023
Revised: 25 July 2023
Accepted: 28 July 2023
Published: 29 July 2023

1. Introduction

Atopic dermatitis (AD), which is also known as atopic eczema, is a skin disorder with a prevalence rate of 15–20% in developed countries [1]. It is usually accompanied by allergic rhinitis, asthma, and infection [2]. Although typically regarded as a childhood disease that presents before children reach one year of age, with the highest prevalence of onset being in 0–6 month-old infants [3], some patients (10–30%) may still have symptoms during adulthood [4]. AD is generally characterized by inflammatory flare-ups accompanied by acute (reddish and swollen) or chronic (lichenified) pruritic lesions on the skin [5]. According to streamlined and validated diagnostic criteria devised by the American Academy of Dermatology (AAD), essential features, such as pruritus, must be present for diagnosis. Some important features, such as an early age of onset, also support the diagnosis [6]. The clinical severity of AD is assessed based on the affected area and intensity using a standardized SCORAD tool [7]. As a recurrent chronic condition, AD affects patients' physical health, financial circumstances, and quality of life [8].

Moisturizers are the mainstay of ongoing management of AD, and topical corticosteroids (TCs) are the first-line treatment for inflammatory symptoms and flare-ups. Topical calcineurin inhibitors (TCIs) are used in tandem with or as alternatives to TCs. In severe cases, systemic therapies, such as systemic corticosteroids, methotrexate, oral cyclosporine, dupilumab, and Janus kinase (JAK) inhibitors, are applied if first-line treatment fails [9,10]. Apart from these therapies, complementary and alternative medicines (CAMs), which are healthcare practices and products, such as herbal remedies, not commonly considered for use in conventional clinical medicine, have also gained popularity among patients with long-term AD who require alternative options to treat their condition [11]. However, these treatment options are used to control AD, decrease symptoms, and reduce flare-ups [12,13], and they cannot cure it. Therefore, creating a management plan is crucial to successful treatment [13].

AD symptom control requires treatment adherence. Poor understanding of the disease, forgetfulness, and the practicalities of applying topical medications have been identified as reasons for non-adherence [14]. Additionally, medications may be misused due to a lack of knowledge about fingertip units (FTU), which describe the quantity of TC to use per application, i.e., an amount from the fingertip to the first crease, that need to be applied to cover a body area the same size as a hand [15]. Also, corticosteroid phobia (corticophobia) is a common cause of treatment non-adherence [16], and it is based on patients' belief that TCs are similar to anabolic or oral steroids [17]. It has also been shown that TCs may lead to adverse reactions, such as skin atrophy, striae distensae, rubeosis, and even adrenal insufficiency, after patients stop their long-term use [18,19]. Moreover, corticophobia could potentially develop in patients due to misinformation presented in the mainstream media [17]. Therefore, better AD symptom control could be achieved by helping patients to understand AD and how to use treatments by giving the right information to patients at the right time.

Since community pharmacists are first-line health providers [20,21], they play a key role in the management of AD, as patients often try over-the-counter treatment before seeking more urgent medical attention [22]. Pharmacists in some jurisdictions, like the UK and USA, can supply low-potency TCs, such as hydrocortisone of up to 1%, without prescriptions, although the majority of treatments are prescribed by specialists or doctors [23,24]. Little information exists regarding the ways in which pharmacists interact with patients regarding AD symptoms or management. More focused and coherent approaches can help pharmacists to support patients with AD, which may improve treatment outcomes. Appropriate counseling could help patients to overcome misinformation and increase adherence, improving symptom control. However, there is no systematic review of the literature regarding the contribution of community pharmacists to the management of AD. Therefore, this systematic review aimed to examine current practices and perceptions of community pharmacists in the management of AD discussed in the literature.

2. Method

2.1. Design

A mixed systematic review was carried out based on a convergent integration approach [25] that used evidence related to practices of community pharmacists and qualitative and quantitative methods.

2.2. Search Strategy

The review followed PRISMA [26] guidelines and was registered with PROSPERO (CRD42022308405). The search strategy, which is explained in the Supplementary Material document (Table S1), identified studies that investigated practices and perceptions of community pharmacists regarding the management of AD. Five databases (Ovid MEDLINE, Ovid EMBASE, EBSCO Cumulative Index to Nursing and Allied Health Literature (CINAHL), PsycINFO, and PubMed) were searched for data collected between their date of inception and December 2022. The search strategy was developed by the primary author (ABC), reviewed by other authors (LL, APR), and quality checked by a specialist librarian.

2.3. Selection Process and Inclusion Criteria

After the search, all identified articles were sent to Endnote. All titles and abstracts were reviewed by ABC to determine their eligibility. All authors assessed these titles against the inclusion criteria, which were determined in line with PICOS (population, intervention, control, outcome, and study design), as shown in Table 1. Inclusion criteria for studies were as follows: (i) research available in full-text form, (ii) primary research discussed in any language, (iii) research published in peer-reviewed journals, and (iv) research that investigated practices and perceptions of community pharmacists regarding the management of AD. Studies that did not fulfil the inclusion criteria were excluded.

Table 1. PICOS.

Population	Patients with atopic dermatitis (all ages)
Intervention	Practices and perceptions of community pharmacists in the management of atopic dermatitis
Control	None
Outcome	Main: Pharmacists' knowledge, recommendations, attitudes, and experiences regarding the management of atopic dermatitis Secondary: Perspectives of others (healthcare providers, patients, and parents) regarding the practices of pharmacists
Study design	Qualitative, quantitative, and mixed methods studies

2.4. Assessment of Methodological Quality

The methodological quality of the studies was appraised by ABC using the Mixed Methods Appraisal Tool (MMAT) [27] and reviewed by the remaining authors (LL, APR). Disagreements were solved via discussion. MMAT was used as it enables quantitative, qualitative, and mixed method studies to be critically appraised [28]. After two screening questions were asked, five questions remained, which participants could answer with either "yes", "no", or "can't tell" responses. The results gave an overall assessment of methodological quality using either 0–1 (low quality), 2–3 (medium quality), or 4–5 (high quality) scores.

2.5. Data Extraction and Synthesis

Information (author and year, country, study design, methods of data collection, participants, number of participants, aim, key findings, and further recommendations of study) was extracted from the involved studies by ABC and reviewed by APR and LL. Data from qualitative and quantitative studies were synthesized using thematic synthesis [29], and a data-based convergent integration approach was applied [25]. Firstly, the quantitative data were subjected to a process known as "qualitizing" or "data transformation", in which quantitative results were turned into textualized qualitative data [30,31]. This process was carried out by ABC, who converted summaries of statistical responses and author commentaries into descriptive textual data, which were then checked by APR and LL to synthetise quantitative data alongside the qualitative findings. Afterwards, the qualitized data and qualitative findings were synthesized via the following three-stage approach: (1) inductive line-by-line coding of findings acquired from themes, quotes, and author commentaries in qualitative studies and descriptive textual data in quantitative and mixed methods studies, as well as author commentaries; (2) combination of related codes into "descriptive" themes; and (3) generation of "analytical" themes based on the interpretation of the findings that went beyond the primary findings [29]. Initial coding and identification of descriptive themes were performed by ABC and reviewed by APR and LL. The agreed descriptive themes were combined into analytical themes through discussion until consensus was achieved among all authors.

2.6. Assessment of Confidence

The confidence of the synthesized findings obtained using qualitized descriptive quantitative and qualitative data was evaluated via the Confidence in the Evidence from Reviews of Qualitative Research (CERQual) tool [32], and findings derived from pre- and post-education intervention studies were assessed using the Grading of Recommendations Assessment, Development, and Evaluation (GRADE) approach [33]. The confidence was assessed using the CERQual tool based on four components—methodological limitations of the included studies, the relevance of included studies to the review question, the coherence of the findings, and the adequacy of the data used to support the review finding—and the GRADE tool was used to evaluate the following criteria: risk of bias, imprecision, inconsistency, indirectness, and magnitude of effect. Both tools judged the quality of evidence using "high", "moderate", "low", or "very low" rankings.

2.7. Outcomes Assessed

The main outcomes assessed to examine practices and perceptions of community pharmacists were their knowledge, recommendations, attitudes, and experiences regarding the management of AD. Secondary outcomes included the perspectives of other individuals (healthcare providers, patients, and parents) on pharmacists' practices.

3. Results

A total of 6657 articles were identified. After removing duplicates and completing the screening stage, 100 studies remained and were evaluated for eligibility, and 80 studies were excluded. A further three studies were identified by searching the references of included studies. Finally, 23 studies (Figure 1), which were all published in English, except for one study published in Japanese, which was translated by a translator, between 1995 and 2021, were included for analysis.

Most studies (n = 19) were conducted in OECD countries: six studies were conducted in the United Kingdom [34–39]; two studies were conducted in each of Australia [40,41], Netherlands [42,43], Sweden [44,45], and Japan [46,47]; and one study was conducted in each of Portugal [48], France [49], Germany [50], Belgium [51], and Italy [52]. Moreover, one study was conducted in a GCC (Gulf Cooperation Council) nation, i.e., the United Arab Emirates [53]. Studies were also carried out in three less developed countries: Jordan [54], South Africa [55], and Iraq [56]. No studies were conducted in the least developed countries.

A majority of studies (n = 20) were published in the period 2011–2021 and reported quantitative findings (n = 18). Of these studies, 14 were cross-sectional studies [37,39,40,46–56] and 4 were pre- and post-education intervention studies [34,41,43,44]. Three were qualitative research [35,42,45]. The remaining studies [36,38] used mixed methods. Table A1 shows a summary of the included studies (see Appendix A section).

The results of quality assessment are shown in Table S2. There was much diversity in scores across studies, which ranged between low and high quality. Only one study was denoted as being of low quality [56]. The quality scores of the quantitative studies ranged from low to high quality, with 13 of 18 studies ranked as being of medium quality. All qualitative studies were ranked as being of high quality [35,42,45]. Two mixed methods studies were rated as being of medium quality [36,38]. Common issues related to study quality and risk of bias for quantitative and mixed methods studies were unclear descriptions of the target population and the sample, as well as well-described inclusion and exclusion criteria for the sample. The main issue that affected qualitative and mixed methods studies was a lack of clarity regarding the way in which the findings were derived from the data.

3.1. Descriptive Themes

Synthesized statements derived from descriptive quantitative and qualitative data were produced, and the confidence level of each statement was assessed using the CERQual tool (see Table S3). Other statements from pre- and post-intervention studies were evaluated using GRADE. As the designs of experimental intervention studies were evaluated as poor, the general rating of findings was reduced from low to very low quality [57]. Two descriptive themes and their sub-themes were identified via the analysis by combining relevant codes (Figure 2; Theme 1: Current Practice and Theme 2: Impact of Pharmacists). The descriptive themes and sub-themes are outlined below.

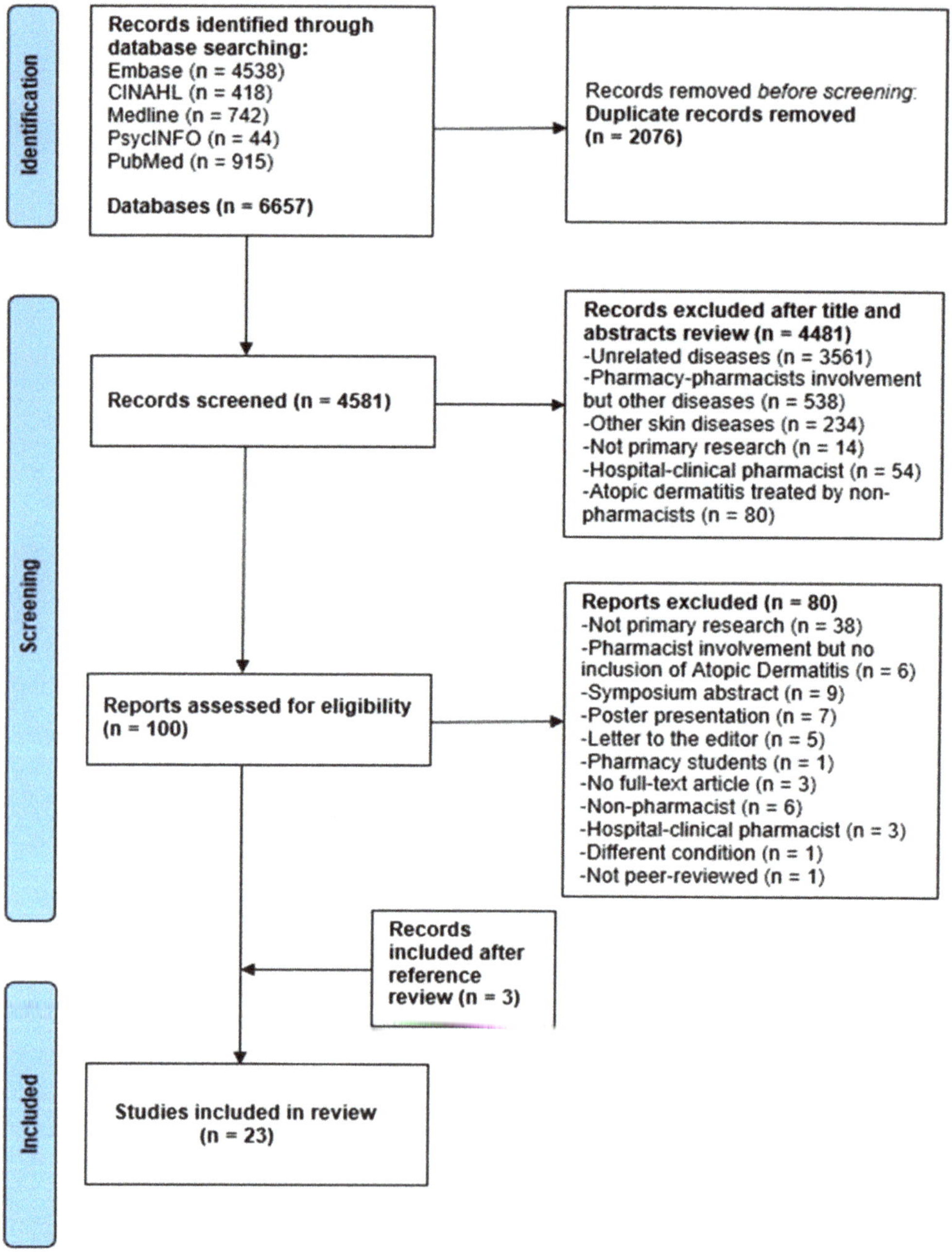

Figure 1. PRISMA flow diagram of search results and included studies.

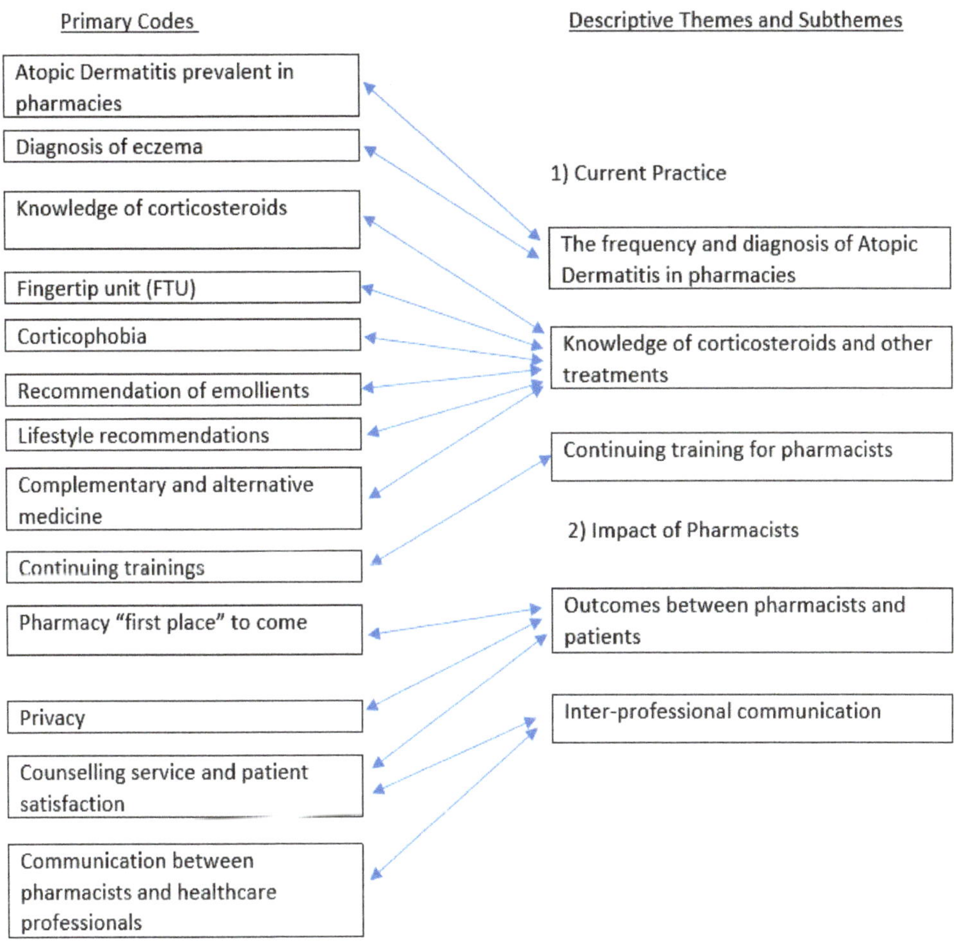

Figure 2. Codes, sub-themes, and descriptive themes.

3.1.1. Current Practice

i. Knowledge of Corticosteroids and Other Treatments

Knowledge of corticosteroids was a significant theme, having FTU- and pharmacist corticophobia-related sub-themes, and it was mentioned in 14 studies [36,41–44,46–54]. Pharmacists were shown to lack knowledge of TC potency in the literature (CERQual-high) [36,53,54]. Poor knowledge regarding the length of TC use was also reported (CERQual-moderate) [48,49,51,54].

Fingertip unit (FTU):

Most pharmacists did not use standard measures, such as FTU, to communicate dosing instructions to patients in the literature. Instead, the literature indicated that patients were told to apply doses thinly (CERQual-moderate) [42,48,54]. Two more studies also stated that a tiny minority of pharmacists recommended FTU to patients (CERQual-moderate) [47,51].

Similarly, pharmacists tended to tell patients to "apply it sparingly" in Australia, though they began using FTU after an educational intervention (GRADE-very low) [41]. It was also found that although most pharmacists knew the amount that can be measured via FTU, only the minority of them often or always advised patients to use this method (CERQual-moderate) [36,47].

Pharmacist corticophobia

Corticophobia was identified in the literature among pharmacists (CERQual-high) [36,42,43,49,51,52]. A Belgian study that compared practitioners found that corticophobia was higher among pharmacists than paediatricians, general practitioners, and dermatologists (CERQual-low) [51]. In France, pharmacists' average confidence regarding corticosteroid use was rated as medium (CERQual-low) [49]. Pharmacists were confused about the side effects of oral corticosteroid and TC use, and they thought that TCs may cause systemic effects (CERQual-moderate) [49,51]. However, it was shown corticophobia can be alleviated via educational intervention (GRADE-very low) [43].

Other treatments, including emollients, lifestyle habit changes, TCIs, and CAMs, were also mentioned [36,42,44,46,54,55]. Regarding emollients, most pharmacists recommended using them as an initial treatment (CERQual-moderate) [36,54], even if they were not prescribed by doctors (CERQual-low) [42], and patients were advised by pharmacists to use them regularly for a prolonged period (CERQual-low) [36]. CAM use was mentioned in only one study [55] and CAMs were seen as more comprehensive and beneficial treatments than current treatment by some pharmacists (CERQual-low). Recommendation of TCI use was mentioned in one study, in which pharmacists explained that a tingling sensation is a common side effect about which patients should not worry (CERQual-low) [46]. Another study noted that pharmacists rarely gave recommendations about lifestyle habits to patients (CERQual-low) [42].

ii. The Frequency and Diagnosis of Atopic Dermatitis in Pharmacies

AD is one of the most prevalent skin conditions seen in pharmacies (CERQual-moderate) [37,39,40,48]. Community pharmacists carry out more medicine reviews for eczema than any other skin condition in the UK (CERQual-low) [39].

Two studies evaluated the diagnostic ability of pharmacists using expert assessors [38,40]. Although some assessors concurred with the diagnoses determined by pharmacists, medical history-recording behaviors of pharmacists were found to be inadequate (CERQual-low) [38]. Furthermore, only in 67% of cases diagnosed as AD did a dermatologist agree with a pharmacist's decision (CERQual-low) [40].

iii. Continuing Training for Pharmacists

Many studies demonstrated that pharmacists often continued their dermatology education after graduation (CERQual-moderate) [36,37,39,40,49,52,53,55]. Pharmacists were eager to expand their dermatological expertise, which they acquired by joining educational programs or training sessions held by drug manufacturers, attending conferences and branch meetings, or reading journal articles and e-bulletins (CERQual-moderate) [35–37,49]. There was a strong correlation between the extent to which continuing their training in dermatology helped pharmacists and their overall self-confidence (CERQual-low) [39]. Pharmacists who undertook continued dermatology training displayed better knowledge, attitude, and practices regarding TC treatment (CERQual-moderate) [53].

3.1.2. Impact of Pharmacists

i. Outcomes between Pharmacists and Patients

Three sub-themes were identified in the literature as being associated with outcomes between pharmacists and patients: "pharmacy first place to come", "counseling service", and "privacy" [34,37,38,41,43–45,52,54,56]. Some studies placed emphasis on pharmacies as the first place that patients visit upon developing a skin problem (CERQual-high) [37,45,52,54], though patients were referred to doctors if they had flare-ups or the condition deteriorated (CERQual-moderate) [45,54].

Counseling services by pharmacists were also reported [34,37,38,43,44,52,56], and most patients were satisfied with the service (GRADE-very low) [34,43], as were pharmacists (GRADE-very low) [44]. However, in a study conducted in Iraq, most patients did not receive any information about the use and adverse effects of TCs from pharmacists (CERQual-very low) [56].

Patient privacy was not usually a concern for pharmacists [41,45]. Pharmacists held consultations with patients in front of other people (GRADE-very low) [41], and patients reported feeling agitated during the consultation [45]. Furthermore, patients reported that pharmacists were not able to understand patients' circumstances (CERQual-low) [45].

ii. Inter-professional Communication

In the literature, communication and collaboration between pharmacists and healthcare professionals was weak (CERQual-moderate) [35,45,49,50]. For example, different guidelines were used by healthcare professionals, with no synchronized approach used, and this issue may cause confusion for patients (CERQual-low) [35]. Moreover, the duration of use of TCs prescribed by physicians was mostly decreased by pharmacists after plausibility checks (CERQual-moderate) [49,50].

3.2. Analytical Themes

Through the analysis of descriptive themes, two analytical themes were determined, which sought to go beyond the findings reported in the original study [58]. The analytical themes discovered were "misleading position" and "perceptions of education and training".

3.2.1. Misleading Position

Pharmacists potentially misinformed patients regarding knowledge of and recommendations and practices regarding AD and its treatment. Although AD was a skin condition commonly seen in pharmacies, while community pharmacists considered themselves to be first-line providers of treatment to patients with dermatologic conditions (Quote 1), they may misinform patients using TCs because of their insufficient knowledge about the potency of TCs (Quote 2).

> *"Pharmacists should be the first port of call for patients with a skin problem".* [37] Quote 1

> *"In terms of formulations, over 60% did not know how many topical corticosteroid potency categories exist".* [36] Quote 2

Besides insufficient knowledge of TCs, pharmacists lacked a standardized way of communicating advice to patients who used topical treatments. Rather than using FTU, they recommended thinly applying topical medications (Quote 3).

> *"Of course, you have those fingertip units. Well, I must confess that we don't really work with it to indicate how much you have to apply. We just say: apply thin. It is still a hormone cream".* [42] Quote 3 (Pharmacist)

Moreover, different terms, besides "applying thinly", were used by pharmacists, which may make patients more confused and worsen existing corticophobia. Subsequently, this situation may result in treatment non-adherence.

> *"When directing the amount of TCS to be applied, 54% reported informing the patient that TCS should be used sparingly..."* [41] Quote 4

Despite AD being one of the most commonly encountered conditions in pharmacies, the pharmacists' ability to record medical histories in some cases was poor (Quote 5). This issue may lead to patients being misinformed about the proper use of treatment or cause misdiagnosis.

> *"A more detailed history would have been helpful and may have supported making the diagnosis".* [38] Quote 5 (Dermatology Specialists)

Regarding emollients, although pharmacists advised patients to apply emollients, even if they were not prescribed (Quote 6), they did not take into consideration the utility of tailored moisturizers for different skin types, sensitivities, or allergies.

> *"Maybe they weren't told about the emollient at the GP. And then you give the advice to use a moisturizer..."* [42] Quote 6 (Pharmacist)

Overall, with moderate-to-high confidence, the evidence suggests that pharmacists were misinforming patients about AD management in practice. With lower confidence, findings also suggested poor diagnosis by pharmacists. Therefore, we can conclude with moderate confidence that community pharmacists may inadvertently play a role in patients being misdiagnosed, inaccurately using treatment, or using an insufficient amount of medicine.

3.2.2. Perceptions of Education and Training

The literature showed that pharmacists received postgraduate training in dermatology, and most appeared to be satisfied with these educational tools. Besides training, pharmacists and their teams used educational interventions for the treatment of AD, which helped them to improve their treatment practices (Quote 7,8).

> *"Of those (pharmacists) surveyed, 92% stated they would advise TCS be used until the eczema is clear, compared to 27% prior to education (p < 0.0001)".* [41] Quote 7

> *"Knowledge about eczema and treatment among pharmacy staff increased from baseline to follow-up 7.3 ± 1.7 to 8.4 ± 1.5 (p = 0.052)".* [43] Quote 8

Furthermore, the pharmacists who attended educational training sessions or interventions could better counsel patients, which resulted in improvements in the management of the condition (Quote 9).

> *"Also, parents were, in general, positive about the counseling session in the pharmacy [. . .] 45.8% mentioned they started using the treatment differently afterwards (e.g., more frequent use of emollients and increased application of TCS, based on FTU)".* [43] Quote 9

Considering the educational level of community pharmacists regarding dermatology, further educational training is perceived as effective at improving practice and patient care. However, in the literature, current practice of pharmacists was poor, which may be caused by the fact that knowledge acquired via initial education alone might not be enough to ensure good quality care in practice. Hence, the gap between pharmacists' knowledge and the needs of the patients can be addressed by improving dermatological education in the initial training of pharmacists.

Overall, with moderate confidence, the evidence showed that pharmacists were willing to extend their knowledge through further education, though the confidence of findings regarding the effectiveness of educational interventions was very low.

4. Discussion

4.1. Summary of Findings

This study reviewed the literature regarding the practices and perceptions of community pharmacists in the management of AD. A key treatment recommended by pharmacists was TCs, though only a few studies mentioned their knowledge and practices regarding other treatments. The most striking finding to emerge from the analysis is that pharmacists did not effectively communicate information about TCs to patients. Pharmacists lacked knowledge of TC practice and duration of treatment. In addition, they had corticophobia. Although most pharmacists knew about FTU, they did not use it. Even though "apply thin" has been removed from labels and the FTU has been promoted in the Netherlands since 2013 [59], this practice was retained by pharmacists in 2019 [42].

Regarding corticophobia, some pharmacists exhibited more fear of using TCs than other healthcare professionals, and this situation encouraged patients to be suspicious of TCs. A key finding is that a pharmacist's stance on TCs may mislead patients regarding their effective use and treatment. A similar position was offered by Smith et al., who reported that cautious approach preferred by pharmacists may encourage patients to avoid TCs [60]. Subsequently, this situation may lead to the ineffectiveness of therapy, since corticophobia is already quite high in patients with AD from 15 different countries [61] and seen as one of the main reasons for non-adherence [16]. It cannot be denied that corticophobia is common in patients; however, it is important for pharmacists to provide accurate and unbiased information and support to patients with AD.

Another key finding is that pharmacists could provide better AD support in practice if they received more comprehensive education on dermatology. It was shown that the counseling practice of community pharmacists was affected by their level of education [62]. This finding is supported by a previous study, which found that re-education of pharmacists was a potential way to enhance confidence in the treatment provided [60], especially as the ability to address dermatological questions has been found to be low among pharmacy students [63]. In addition, receiving educational training was linked to confidence in dealing with skin conditions [64]. Furthermore, an e-learning educational program that included corticophobia and FTU sections was implemented in a past study, and an increase in the knowledge of AD management was observed in pharmacists [65].

4.2. Implications for Practice and Policy

While community pharmacists play a key role in counseling patients with AD, they lacked practical knowledge of the management of the condition. Pharmacists could negatively influence patients by advising incorrect ways of using topical treatments, preventing proper use of TCs and potentially causing misdiagnosis of conditions. The findings also showed that pharmacists attended a range of training courses related to dermatology after graduation. There is an evident gap between patient needs in pharmacy practice and initial education. This gap can potentially be reduced via educational interventions, such as giving pharmacy students sufficient knowledge of the use of TCs and other topical treatments and providing more comprehensive competency-based practice education regarding dermatology. If patients are not appropriately helped to manage their condition by pharmacists, they may continue their usual routine, and the condition may remain unmanaged. An increase in the number of unmanaged AD patients may put more financial burden on countries' health systems, since AD has a significant financial effect on health care systems [66]. To avoid this burden, preventative action can be taken by policymakers and academics. Providing dermatological training during initial pharmacy education should help pharmacists to develop the improved knowledge and skills required to meet patients' needs in practice. This training should draw on expertise from dermatologists, patient experts, and practices that are captured in current guidance [23,67,68]. This training needs to be ongoing and embedded in practice through continuous professional development to ensure that pharmacists can appropriately assess, diagnose, prescribe, and monitor AD, as well as communicate with patients, in community pharmacy settings.

4.3. Strengths and Limitations of the Study

The strength of the study is that it identified, for the first time, the current strengths and weaknesses of the practices used by pharmacists to supporting patients with AD. Regarding limitations, TC was the most commonly mentioned medication in this review, though it does not give a full picture of counseling practices used by pharmacists for all treatment options. Some studies notably concentrated on paediatric eczema, though eczema is not seen in children alone. Some included studies discussed other skin conditions besides AD, and this issue may limit these studies' findings' of relevance to AD. In addition, all studies were derived from either OECD, GCC, or less developed countries; thus, the findings of this study may not be applicable to least developed countries. Some studies cited other healthcare professionals as well as pharmacists, and it was possible to separate the findings attributed to pharmacists in these studies. However, in two studies [43,44], pharmacists and technicians, and in one study, [46] community and hospital pharmacists were grouped together as pharmacy staff, meaning that distinguishing the pharmacists' contributions was not possible in these studies.

4.4. Further Research

Further studies are needed to broaden this topic's focus to cover other treatments of AD, rather than only studying TCs. The focus of future pedagogical research needs to be on establishing steps that can be taken as part of initial education to improve practice of future pharmacists in supporting patients with AD. Based on the low confidence rates presented in some studies, more robust research is needed. There is also a gap in evidence regarding pharmacist management of AD in least developed countries.

5. Conclusions

The purpose of the study was to examine community pharmacists' contribution to the management of AD. This study has shown a gap between community pharmacy practice and pharmacists' training and education. This gap means that pharmacists inadvertently mislead patients in practice by reinforcing fear of TC use and providing inadequate counseling about the duration and application of topical treatment. Despite significant receiving undergraduate and postgraduate training, the literature indicates that community pharmacists lacked the knowledge and skills required to effectively respond to the needs of AD patients in practice, encouraging them to seek further dermatology training to make up for the educational deficiency of their initial training. The findings of this research provide insights into the gap between practice and education, showing that novel educational interventions are required to improve AD management.

Supplementary Materials: The following supporting information can be downloaded at: https://www.mdpi.com/article/10.3390/healthcare11152159/s1, Table S1: Detailed search strategy; Table S2: Quality assessment of included studies; Table S3: CERQual full evidence profile; File S1: PRISMA 2020 checklist. Refs [26,34–56] are cited in Supplementary Materials.

Author Contributions: Conceptualization, A.B.C., A.P.R. and L.L.; validation, A.B.C., A.P.R. and L.L.; formal analysis, A.B.C., A.P.R. and L.L.; investigation and resources, A.B.C., A.P.R. and L.L.; data curation, A.B.C., A.P.R. and L.L.; writing—original draft preparation, A.B.C.; writing—review and editing, A.B.C., A.P.R. and L.L.; visualization, A.B.C.; supervision, A.P.R. and L.L.; project administration, A.B.C.; funding acquisition, A.B.C. All authors have read and agreed to the published version of the manuscript.

Funding: The APC was funded by Newcastle University Open Access funding.

Institutional Review Board Statement: Not applicable.

Informed Consent Statement: Not applicable.

Data Availability Statement: Data that support the reported findings of this study are found in the Ovid MEDLINE, Ovid EMBASE, EBSCO Cumulative Index to Nursing and Allied Health Literature (CINAHL), PsycINFO, and PubMed databases.

Acknowledgments: This work was conducted as a part of a doctoral study, supported and funded by the Ministry of National Education of the Republic of Türkiye.

Conflicts of Interest: The authors declare no conflict of interest.

Appendix A

Table A1. Summary of included studies.

Author and Year	Country	Study Design	Methods of Data Collection	Participants	Number of Participants	Aim	Key Findings	Further Recommendations
Abed et al. [56], 2021	Iraq	Cross-sectional	Questionnaire	Customers who asked for topical corticosteroids (TCs) without prescription	212 customers	To assess the patients' knowledge of TC use and education provided by pharmacists	• The lack of pharmacist practice regarding patient education	• Health officials should raise awareness of incorrect use of TCs by advertising in public and via traditional and social media.
Carr et al. [34], 2009	England	Pre-post educational intervention	Questionnaire	Patients and their parents	50 children and their parents	To identify the effects of community pharmacists' interventions on the use of emollients in children with eczema	• Pharmacists' interventions reduced some symptoms to a moderate yet significant extent. In addition, the intervention taught patients to apply emollients properly. • Although intervention was found to be useful, it requires pharmacists that devote a lot of time; thus, s new pharmacy regulations may make it easier for pharmacists to counsel patients.	• The small number of pharmacies referenced in this study may not reflect the aspect of all pharmacists and some of them in this study have experience of offering counseling services. Therefore, this study may give inaccurate outcomes. To conclude, a greater number of pharmacies should be included for next studies.
Cowdell et al. [35], 2019	England	Qualitative study	Field notes and interviews	Community pharmacists and other health professionals	2 community pharmacists	To create positive atopic dermatitis (AD)-related mindsets among healthcare practitioners to improve management of the condition	• Eczema was seen as simple condition to treat by practitioners, and they thought eczema treatment has changed little over time. Therefore, they did not need to improve their knowledge. However, pharmacy staff increased their knowledge through formal and informal sources.	• Outdated mindsets should be removed by introducing reliable and beneficial knowledge. Improving mindsets is crucial for self-management of AD.
Giua et al. [52], 2021	Italy	Cross-sectional	Questionnaire	Community pharmacists	154 community pharmacists	(1) To obtain information about pharmacists' counseling activity regarding dermatological conditions; (2) to gain information about corticophobia among pharmacists; (3) to research the educational needs of pharmacists	• AD was the most known of all dermatitis types by pharmacists (79.9%). • Pharmacists generally provided counseling services to all patients at least once a week. • A majority of pharmacists (57.1%) believed that patients visit pharmacies before seeing a doctor. • Although most of pharmacists (66.9%) thought that patients were adherent, they underestimated corticosteroid phobia (corticophobia) between patients, as only a minority of them had positive opinions about topical corticosteroids.	• Pharmacists think that educational tools would be beneficial to solve the knowledge gap.

Table A1. *Cont.*

Author and Year	Country	Study Design	Methods of Data Collection	Participants	Number of Participants	Aim	Key Findings	Further Recommendations
Hammarstrom et al. [44], 1995	Sweden	Pre-post educational intervention	Questionnaire and drug sale statistics	Community pharmacies	900 community pharmacies	To improve treatment management in patients with skin disorders	• Almost all pharmacy staff agreed that input from local pharmacies in improving treatment of skin disorders was substantial. • Both over-the-counter (OTC) and prescribed medication use significantly increased after campaign was held. • The highest increase was recorded regarding the use of emollients. • The increase in use of corticosteroids resulted from the campaign in which pharmacists emphasized importance of corticosteroid use in the management of AD. • It was obvious that a transition from prescribed to non-prescribed medication use was seen after the campaign.	• It is important to introduce more campaigns among community pharmacies.
Issa et al. [54], 2016	Jordan	Cross-sectional	Questionnaire	Community pharmacists	100 community pharmacists	To evaluate the disagreements in TCs prescription patterns and practice advices among different health workers and determine underlying causes	• Pharmacists lacked knowledge about the potency of topical corticosteroids. • Most pharmacists (67%) recommended "apply thin" instead of using "fingertip unit (FTU)" regarding use of topical corticosteroids. • Despite the fact that a large majority of pharmacists (68%) recommended that patients see doctor in case of flare-ups, 28% of them still suggested the use of mid-high- or high-dose corticosteroids. • Just over a third of pharmacists (36%) suggested the use of emollients for patients with mild eczema.	• It is important to update pharmacists regarding practice guidelines to develop effective AD treatment.
Jairoun et al. [53], 2020	United Arab Emirates	Cross-sectiona	Questionnaire	Community pharmacists	772 community pharmacists	To find out pharmacist knowledge, attitude, and practice in use of corticosteroids	• Pharmacists with more experience had better knowledge and used better practices regarding corticosteroids. • Pharmacists who received educational training had better questionnaire scores than those who did not receive training. • There were knowledge, attitude, and practice differences between those who graduated from international and local institutions. • There was low score in terms of use of potent corticosteroid in cases of acute flare ups of eczema. • Many pharmacists thought that corticosteroids should not be used in children.	• Proper courses regarding the appropriate use of corticosteroids should be integrated into the curriculum to educate pharmacists.

Table A1. *Cont.*

Author and Year	Country	Study Design	Methods of Data Collection	Participants	Number of Participants	Aim	Key Findings	Further Recommendations
Kaneko et al. [46], 2014	Japan	Cross-sectional	Questionnaire	Community and hospital pharmacists	372 community, 109 hospital pharmacists	To investigate pharmacist practices regarding applying topical medications in the management of AD	• Pharmacists mainly explained the best application site to patients regarding use of corticosteroids if they were using it first time, and pharmacists' knowledge of guidelines positively affected their recommendations. • Pharmacists urged patients to apply topical medications until their situation improved. • Pharmacists gave information about tingling effects associated with the use of calcineurin inhibitors and told patients that this issue is common side effect. However, this approach caused anxiety in some patients. • Pharmacists complained that doctors' instructions regarding the frequency and site of application were not clear.	To effectively counsel eczema patients, pharmacists should be aware of treatment guidelines for AD and are urged to follow these guidelines.
Koster et al. [42], 2019	Netherlands	Qualitative study	Interviews	Parents of children with AD, community pharmacists and pharmacy technicians	29 parents, 6 community pharmacists, and 12 pharmacy technicians	To explore the perspectives of both pharmacy staff and parents regarding the treatment of children with AD in the Netherlands	• Pharmacists thought patients suddenly gave up corticosteroid, which was caused by the fact that pharmacy staff give misinformed information about corticosteroid use, which led to corticophobia in patients. • Pharmacists did not use FTU to indicate the amount of cream that patients should apply. They simply told patients to thinly apply the cream. • Pharmacists recommended the use of emollients in addition to treatment, even if they were not prescribed. • Parents of children with AD needed additional information about lifestyle habits from pharmacists.	• The problem of insufficient practical skills and knowledge about AD among pharmacy staff needs to be rectified.
Koster et al. [43], 2021	Netherlands	Pre- and post-education interventions	Questionnaire	Parents of children with AD, community pharmacists, and pharmacy technicians	48 parents, 6 community pharmacists, and 13 pharmacy technicians	To study the effects of pharmacy intervention on corticophobia among both pharmacy staff and parents of young AD patients	• Educational interventions may be useful to overcome corticophobia, which is measured via the TOPICOP scale, for both pharmacy staff and parents of children with AD. • The corticophobia score of pharmacy staff significantly decreased from 33.2 to 25.1% between pre- and post-intervention test. • Knowledge of pharmacy staff about eczema and treatment rose after educational intervention. • Parents of patients were happy with counseling serviced and began using medicines more regularly. • Patients' eczema conditions improved substantially after they received counseling services.	• The follow-up time was short, meaning that it could only provide information about short-term effects of the intervention. Pharmacy staff should be regularly trained to provide optimal treatment to patients.

Table A1. *Cont.*

Author and Year	Country	Study Design	Methods of Data Collection	Participants	Number of Participants	Aim	Key Findings	Further Recommendations
Lambrechts et al. [51], 2019	Belgium	Cross-sectional	Questionnaire	Pharmacists, paediatricians, GPs, dermatologists	118 pharmacists, 100 paediatricians, 81 GPs, and 92 dermatologists.	To determine the frequency of corticophobia among pharmacists and other health professionals	• Pharmacists made up the group with the highest rate of corticophobia all other health professionals. • More than half of pharmacists (55.1%) had proper knowledge of the amount that should be applied, and about half of them (48.3%) knew that a corticosteroid medicine must be used until eczema disappears. • A minority of pharmacists (21.2%) recommended FTU as the best method with regard to the use of TCs.	• Corticophobia among health professionals remains an issue because of insufficient knowledge, meaning that staff should be further trained, as approximately one-third of pharmacists do not remember receiving courses about TCs
Lau et al. [36], 2017	England	Mixed-methods	Interviews and questionnaire	Community pharmacists	5 community pharmacists were interviewed and 105 community pharmacists filled out the questionnaire.	To investigate the knowledge of community pharmacists regarding corticosteroid use in the treatment of AD, as well as their information supply, attitudes, and patient counseling behavior	• Some pharmacists (36.2%) received extra postgraduate training related to dermatology. • Most pharmacists (62.9%) inaccurately categorized corticosteroids in terms of their potency. • Regarding corticosteroids, a minority of pharmacists stated that if patients use them correctly, side effects are not common. • Though most of them (90.5%) knew about FTU, only a third of pharamcists (36.2%) always or often recommended this method when counseling patients. • Pharmacists had more knowledge of the use of emollients than corticosteroids.	• Pharmacists perceptions of corticosteroid safety are low. They need to be improved to ensure that they can effectively counsel patients.
Lindblad et al. [45], 2006	Sweden	Qualitative	Focus groups	Patients and health providers (community pharmacists, dermatology nurses, and dermatologists)	12 patients and 12 health providers (the number of pharmacists was not applicable)	To determine the views of health providers and patients regarding the role of providers in the management of derma-tological conditions	• If patients have not yet seen a doctor and do not know about their situation, pharmacists gave them basic information about eczema and some weak corticosteroids. • Health providers labelled pharmacists as having "initial screener" and "final checker" roles. However, there is a lack of collaboration between pharmacists, nurses, and doctors. • Patients thought that pharmacists lacked understanding of their situations and claimed that there was lack of privacy in pharmacies, and they did not feel able to communicate with pharmacists.	• There is a need for successful cooperation between pharmacists and other health providers. Pharmacists suggest that regular meetings can be held regarding finding medicine information to settle the conflict. In addition, some strategies should be implemented to embed dermatology in healthcare systems.

Table A1. *Cont.*

Author and Year	Country	Study Design	Methods of Data Collection	Participants	Number of Participants	Aim	Key Findings	Further Recommendations
Manahan et al. [40], 2011	Australia	Cross-sectional	Questionnaire	Community pharmacists and pharmacy interns	17 community pharmacists and 3 pharmacy interns	To identify community pharmacists' roles in the management of skin conditions and assess their opinions of teledermatology services	• Almost half of cases managed by pharmacists were eczema. • In 2/3 of cases diagnosed as eczema, a dermatologist completely agreed with the pharmacist's management of the condition. • All pharmacists were keen to received further education related to dermatology.	• A system of pharmacist–tele dermatologist cooperation could improve the management of diseases and alleviate the burden on GPs.
Oishi et al. [47], 2019	Japan	Cross-sectional	Questionnaire	Community pharmacists	300 community pharmacists	To investigate the effectiveness of community pharmacists' instructions regarding the use of FTU and the effects of following practice guidelines on treatment	• A small minority of pharmacists (14.3%) always used FTU to the primary method of corticosteroid application. • The level of comprehension of best practice guidelines correlated with pharmacists' ability to give instructions about topical corticosteroid use. • Though pharmacists considered corticosteroid application amounts and sites, the timing of doses was ignored.	• Community pharmacists must be acquainted with best practice guidelines to ensure that they can counsel patients about their treatment.
Raffin et al. [49], 2016	France	Cross-sectional	Questionnaire	Community pharmacists technicians and students	176 community pharmacists, 10 pharmacy technicians, and 5 pharmacy students	To evaluate corticophobia among pharmacists in relation to AD in children	• Among pharmacists, there was lack of knowledge about side effects of corticosteroids admiistered via topical and oral applications. • Pharamcists had a lack of information about duration of corticosteroid treatment. • Opposing instructions from pharmacists and physicians can cause confusion and fear in patients. • A vast majority of pharmacists wanted to receive education about AD in children.	• Continuing training for pharmacists regarding the use of corticosteroids is recommended to improve adherence results.
Salzmann et al. [50], 2020	Germany	Cross-sectional	Questionnaire	Community pharmacists and dermatologists	351 community pharmacists and 53 dermatologists	To acquire data about daily prescription habits related to compounded preparations (CPs) in dermatology and compare them using standardized questionnaires, as well as to overcome the lack of interdisciplinary collaboration	• Pharmacists viewed compounded preparations as an "important treatment alternative". • There was inadequate communication and collaboration between pharmacists and dermatologists.	Future studies should concentrate on CPs to increase the quality of prescriptions.

Table A1. *Cont.*

Author and Year	Country	Study Design	Methods of Data Collection	Participants	Number of Participants	Aim	Key Findings	Further Recommendations
Smith et al. [41], 2016	Australia	Pre-post educational intervention	Survey	Pharmacists (including community pharmacists)	292 pharmacists	To evaluate pharmacists' beliefs and knowledge regarding the use of topical corticosteroids in paediatric eczema	• The proportion of pharmacists who talked to patients separately for privacy reasons significantly increased from 41 to 78%. • The share of pharmacists who recommended applying treatments as shown on prescription rose from 52 to 88%. • The proportion of those who suggested corticosteroid use until eczema cleared up rose to 92%, and those who suggested a maximum use period of one week declined to 2%. • The percentage of pharmacists who told patients to apply treatments sparingly fell to 8%.	Pharmacist education throughout initial education and pharmacy journals should be supported by dermatology specialists to enhance pharmacists' knowledge of the use of TCs in AD.
Teixeira et al. [48], 2021	Portugal	Cross-sectional	Questionnaire	Community pharmacists and patients	149 community pharmacists, 44 patients	To find the association between pharmacists' knowledge and their conveyance of information to patients with dermatoses and create a proper guide for patients about dosage instructions	• Atopic dermatitis (84.3%) was the most prevalent condition in Portugal according to pharmacists. • 63.9% of pharmacists thought that they always provided information about the duration of treatment with topical corticosteroids. • 50% of pharmacists always instructed patients on how to apply medicine, and 85.2% of phramacists instructed patients on how to "apply in thin layer" while applying a topical medicine.	Proper guidelines must be prepared to enhance communication of dosage instructions to patients. Moreover, continued training courses should be implemented to help pharmacists to solve problems.
Thandar et al. [55], 2019	South Africa	Cross-sectional	Questionnaire	Community pharmacists	82 community pharmacists	To identify community pharmacists' attitudes and practices regarding the use of complementary and alternative therapies in patients with AD	• More than a third of pharmacists (35%) thought that complementary and alternative medicines (CAMs) outweighed conventional therapy in terms of effectiveness. • Almost all pharmacists supported including CAMs in university curriculums. • Although most pharmacists were not acquainted with homeopathy and Chinese herbal medicine, they were mostly familiar with probiotics.	It was revealed that pharmacists had insufficient knowledge of CAMs, meaning that they needed further ongoing education.
Tucker et al. [37], 2012	England and Wales	Cross-sectional	Questionnaire	Community Pharmacists	870 community pharmacists	To find out which types of skin diseases pharmacists come across in pharmacies and which training sessions they attend to gain more knowledge of dermatological diseases	• Eczema was the most commonly encountered condition for which patient want advice, besides dry skin complaints. • Most pharmacists (64.8%) received some postgraduate training related to dermatology. • Pharmacists were aware that they have critical roles in counseling patients and should be the first point-of-contact for patients with skin problems.	Use of pharmacists' advice in the management of skin conditions should be studied in future studies.

Table A1. *Cont.*

Author and Year	Country	Study Design	Methods of Data Collection	Participants	Number of Participants	Aim	Key Findings	Further Recommendations
Tucker et al. [39], 2013	England and Wales	Cross-sectional	Questionnaire	Community Pharmacists	870 community pharmacists	To identify pharmacists' roles in medicine use review (MUR) and evaluate pharmacists' understanding of long-term skin diseases	• The most commonly conducted MUR services were in performed patients with eczema. • Pharmacists mostly found postgraduate training to be helpful in terms of dealing with patient requests, and this willingness was positively associated with overall self-confidence.	Further studies should be conducted to identify whether these reviews contribute to better disease-related outcomes.
Tucker et al. [38], 2017	England	Mixed methods	Questionnaire- and assessment-based feedback	Patients, dermatology specialists, and community pharmacists	40 patients, 3 dermatology specialists, and 9 community pharmacists	To assess the clinical convenience of pharmacists' diagnoses and management of dermatitis and acne, as well as to obtain patients' self-reported perceptions regarding the effectiveness of pharmacy intervention	• Pharmacists' diagnoses were evaluated by assessors and found to be accurate in over a third of cases (34%). However, assessors' rate of disagreement with pharmacists' diagnoses was higher. In addition, assessors found the questioning and medica history-recording practices of pharmacists to be inadequate. • Pharmacists' approaches to treatment were accurate in almost half of all cases. • Over half of patients felt that their skin problem had been completely resolved through the treatment provided at the pharmacy.	Patient assessment-related education for pharmacists should be considered, with particuar focus on dermatology.

AD, atopic dermatitis; TCs, topical corticosteroids; OTC, over-the-counter; FTU, fingertip unit; TOPICOP, topical corticosteroid phobia; GP, general practitioner; CPs, compounded preparations, CAMs, complementary and alternative medicines; MUR, medicine use review.

References

1. Weidinger, S.; Beck, L.A.; Bieber, T.; Kabashima, K.; Irvine, A.D. Atopic dermatitis. *Nat. Rev. Dis. Primers* **2018**, *4*, 1–20. [CrossRef]
2. Bekić, S.; Martinek, V.; Talapko, J.; Majnarić, L.; Vasilj Mihaljević, M.; Škrlec, I. Atopic Dermatitis and Comorbidity. *Healthcare* **2020**, *8*, 70. [CrossRef] [PubMed]
3. Kay, J.; Gawkrodger, D.J.; Mortimer, M.J.; Jaron, A.G. The prevalence of childhood atopic eczema in a general population. *J. Am. Acad. Dermatol.* **1994**, *30*, 35–39. [CrossRef] [PubMed]
4. Ellis, C.N.; Mancini, A.J.; Paller, A.S.; Simpson, E.L.; Eichenfield, L.F. Understanding and managing atopic dermatitis in adult patients. *Semin. Cutan. Med. Surg.* **2012**, *31*, S18–S22. [CrossRef] [PubMed]
5. Girolomoni, G.; de Bruin-Weller, M.; Aoki, V.; Kabashima, K.; Deleuran, M.; Puig, L.; Bansal, A.; Rossi, A.B. Nomenclature and clinical phenotypes of atopic dermatitis. *Ther. Adv. Chronic Dis.* **2021**, *12*, 1–20. [CrossRef] [PubMed]
6. Eichenfield, L.F.; Tom, W.L.; Chamlin, S.L.; Feldman, S.R.; Hanifin, J.M.; Simpson, E.L.; Berger, T.G.; Bergman, J.N.; Cohen, D.E.; Cooper, K.D. Guidelines of care for the management of atopic dermatitis: Section 1. Diagnosis and assessment of atopic dermatitis. *J. Am. Acad. Dermatol.* **2014**, *70*, 338–351. [CrossRef]
7. Schallreuter, K.; Levenig, C.; Berger, J.; Umbert, J.; Winkelmann, R.; Wegener, L.; Correia, O.; Chosidow, O.; Saiag, P.; Bastuji-Garin, S. Severity scoring of atopic dermatitis: The SCORAD index. *Dermatology* **1993**, *186*, 23–31.
8. Ng, M.S.; Tan, S.; Chan, N.H.; Foong, A.Y.; Koh, M.J. Effect of atopic dermatitis on quality of life and its psychosocial impact in Asian adolescents. *Australas. J. Dermatol.* **2018**, *59*, e114–e117. [CrossRef]
9. Maliyar, K.; Sibbald, C.; Pope, E.; Sibbald, R.G. Diagnosis and management of atopic dermatitis: A review. *Adv. Ski. Wound Care* **2018**, *31*, 538–550. [CrossRef]
10. Chovatiya, R.; Paller, A.S. JAK inhibitors in the treatment of atopic dermatitis. *J. Allergy Clin. Immunol.* **2021**, *148*, 927–940 [CrossRef]
11. Holm, J.G.; Clausen, M.-L.; Agner, T.; Thomsen, S.F. Use of complementary and alternative therapies in outpatients with atopic dermatitis from a dermatological university department. *Dermatology* **2019**, *235*, 189–195. [CrossRef]
12. Dattola, A.; Bennardo, L.; Silvestri, M.; Nisticò, S.P. What's new in the treatment of atopic dermatitis? *Dermatol. Ther.* **2019**, *32*, e12787. [CrossRef]
13. McAleer, M.; Flohr, C.; Irvine, A. Management of difficult and severe eczema in childhood. *BMJ* **2012**, *345*, e4770. [CrossRef]
14. Patel, N.U.; D'Ambra, V.; Feldman, S.R. Increasing adherence with topical agents for atopic dermatitis. *Am. J. Clin. Dermatol.* **2017**, *18*, 323–332. [CrossRef] [PubMed]
15. Ference, J.D.; Last, A.R. Choosing topical corticosteroids. *Am. Fam. Physician* **2009**, *79*, 135–140.
16. Fischer, G. Compliance problems in paediatric atopic eczema. *Australas. J. Dermatol.* **1996**, *37*, S10–S13. [CrossRef] [PubMed]
17. Charman, C.; Williams, H. The use of corticosteroids and corticosteroid phobia in atopic dermatitis. *Clin. Dermatol.* **2003**, *21*, 193–200. [CrossRef]
18. Niculet, E.; Bobeica, C.; Tatu, A.L. Glucocorticoid-induced skin atrophy: The old and the new. *Clin. Cosmet. Investig. Dermatol.* **2020**, *13*, 1041–1050. [CrossRef]
19. Kijima, T.; Shimada, N.; Ishida, N.; Yamagata, S.; Makiishi, T. Adrenal Insufficiency Following Prolonged Administration of Ultra-High Topical Steroid: A Case of Refractory Dermatitis. *Cureus* **2023**, *15*, e37967. [CrossRef] [PubMed]
20. Roque, F.; Soares, S.; Breitenfeld, L.; López-Durán, A.; Figueiras, A.; Herdeiro, M.T. Attitudes of community pharmacists to antibiotic dispensing and microbial resistance: A qualitative study in Portugal. *Int. J. Clin. Pharm.* **2013**, *35*, 417–424. [CrossRef]
21. Murray, E.; Bieniek, K.; Del Aguila, M.; Egodage, S.; Litzinger, S.; Mazouz, A.; Mills, H.; Liska, J. Impact of pharmacy intervention on influenza vaccination acceptance: A systematic literature review and meta-analysis. *Int. J. Clin. Pharm.* **2021**, *43*, 1163–1172. [CrossRef]
22. Wong, I.T.; Tsuyuki, R.T.; Cresswell-Melville, A.; Doiron, P.; Drucker, A.M. Guidelines for the management of atopic dermatitis (eczema) for pharmacists. *Can. Pharm. J./Rev. Des. Pharm. Du Can.* **2017**, *150*, 285–297. [CrossRef]
23. Atopic Eczema in Under 12s: Diagnosis and Management. National Institute for Health Care Excellence (NICE) Clinical Guideline [CG57]. Available online: https://www.nice.org.uk/guidance/cg57 (accessed on 15 July 2023).
24. Ravis, S.M.; Eaglstein, W.H. Topical hydrocortisone from prescription to over-the-counter sale: A past controversy: A cautionary tale. *Arch. Dermatol.* **2007**, *143*, 413–415. [CrossRef]
25. Pluye, P.; Hong, Q.N. Combining the power of stories and the power of numbers: Mixed methods research and mixed studies reviews. *Annu. Rev. Public Health* **2014**, *35*, 29–45. [CrossRef] [PubMed]
26. Page, M.J.; McKenzie, J.E.; Bossuyt, P.M.; Boutron, I.; Hoffmann, T.C.; Mulrow, C.D.; Shamseer, L.; Tetzlaff, J.M.; Akl, E.A.; Brennan, S.E.; et al. The PRISMA 2020 statement: An updated guideline for reporting systematic reviews. *BMJ* **2021**, *372*, 71. [CrossRef] [PubMed]
27. Hong, Q.N.; Pluye, P.; Fàbregues, S.; Bartlett, G.; Boardman, F.; Cargo, M.; Dagenais, P.; Gagnon, M.-P.; Griffiths, F.; Nicolau, B. *Mixed Methods Appraisal Tool (MMAT)*; Version 2018; Registration of Copyright Canadian Intellectual Property Office, Industry Canada: Gatineau, QC, Canada, 2018.
28. Pace, R.; Pluye, P.; Bartlett, G.; Macaulay, A.C.; Salsberg, J.; Jagosh, J.; Seller, R. Testing the reliability and efficiency of the pilot Mixed Methods Appraisal Tool (MMAT) for systematic mixed studies review. *Int. J. Nurs. Stud.* **2012**, *49*, 47–53. [CrossRef] [PubMed]

29. Thomas, J.; Harden, A. Methods for the thematic synthesis of qualitative research in systematic reviews. *BMC Med. Res. Methodol.* **2008**, *8*, 45. [CrossRef]
30. Sandelowski, M. Combining qualitative and quantitative sampling, data collection, and analysis techniques in mixed-method studies. *Res. Nurs. Health* **2000**, *23*, 246–255. [CrossRef]
31. Hong, Q.N.; Pluye, P.; Bujold, M.; Wassef, M. Convergent and sequential synthesis designs: Implications for conducting and reporting systematic reviews of qualitative and quantitative evidence. *Syst. Rev.* **2017**, *6*, 61. [CrossRef]
32. Lewin, S.; Glenton, C.; Munthe-Kaas, H.; Carlsen, B.; Colvin, C.J.; Gülmezoglu, M.; Noyes, J.; Booth, A.; Garside, R.; Rashidian, A. Using qualitative evidence in decision making for health and social interventions: An approach to assess confidence in findings from qualitative evidence syntheses (GRADE-CERQual). *PLoS Med.* **2015**, *12*, e1001895. [CrossRef]
33. Guyatt, G.H.; Oxman, A.D.; Vist, G.E.; Kunz, R.; Falck-Ytter, Y.; Alonso-Coello, P.; Schünemann, H.J. GRADE: An emerging consensus on rating quality of evidence and strength of recommendations. *BMJ* **2008**, *336*, 924–926. [CrossRef]
34. Carr, A.; Patel, R.; Jones, M.; Suleman, A. A pilot study of a community pharmacist intervention to promote the effective use of emollients in childhood eczema. *Pharm. J.* **2007**, *278*, 319–322.
35. Cowdell, F. Knowledge mobilisation: An ethnographic study of the influence of practitioner mindlines on atopic eczema self-management in primary care in the UK. *BMJ Open* **2019**, *9*, e025220. [CrossRef] [PubMed]
36. Lau, W.M.; Donyai, P. Knowledge, Attitude and Advice-Giving Behaviour of Community Pharmacists Regarding Topical Corticosteroids. *Pharmacy* **2017**, *5*, 41. [CrossRef] [PubMed]
37. Tucker, R. Community pharmacists' perceptions of the skin conditions they encounter and how they view their role in dermatological care. *Int. J. Pharm. Pract.* **2012**, *20*, 344–346. [CrossRef] [PubMed]
38. Tucker, R.P.; MacLure, K.; Paudyal, V.; Layton, A.M.; Bewley, A.; Stewart, D. An exploratory study of community pharmacist diagnosis and management of dermatitis and acne. *Selfcare* **2017**, *8*, 1–10.
39. Tucker, R. The medicines use review in patients with chronic skin diseases: Are pharmacists doing them and how confident are they? *Int. J. Pharm. Pract.* **2013**, *21*, 202–204. [CrossRef] [PubMed]
40. Manahan, M.N.; Soyer, H.P.; Nissen, L.M. Teledermatology in pharmacies: A pilot study. *J. Telemed. Telecare* **2011**, *17*, 392–396. [CrossRef]
41. Smith, S.D.; Lee, A.; Blaszczynski, A.; Fischer, G. Pharmacists' knowledge about use of topical corticosteroids in atopic dermatitis: Pre and post continuing professional development education. *Australas. J. Dermatol.* **2016**, *57*, 199–204. [CrossRef]
42. Koster, E.S.; Philbert, D.; Wagelaar, K.R.; Galle, S.; Bouvy, M.L. Optimizing pharmaceutical care for pediatric patients with dermatitis: Perspectives of parents and pharmacy staff. *Int. J. Clin. Pharm.* **2019**, *41*, 711–718. [CrossRef]
43. Koster, E.S.; Philbert, D.; Zheng, X.; Moradi, N.; de Vries, T.W.; Bouvy, M.L. Reducing corticosteroid phobia in pharmacy staff and parents of children with atopic dermatitis. *Int. J. Clin. Pharm.* **2021**, *43*, 1237–1244. [CrossRef]
44. Hammarström, B.; Wessling, A.; Nilsson, J.L. Pharmaceutical care for patients with skin diseases: A campaign year at Swedish pharmacies. *J. Clin. Pharm. Ther.* **1995**, *20*, 327–334. [CrossRef] [PubMed]
45. Lindblad, A.K.; Kjelgren, K.I.; Ring, L.; Maroti, M.; Serup, J. The role of dermatologists, nurses and pharmacists in chronic dermatological treatment: Patient and provider views and experiences. *Acta Derm. Venereol.* **2006**, *86*, 202–208. [CrossRef]
46. Kaneko, S.; Kakamu, T.; Matsuo, H.; Naora, K.; Morita, E. Questionnaire-based study on the key to the guidance to the patients with atopic dermatitis by pharmacist. *Jpn. J. Allergol.* **2014**, *63*, 1250–1257.
47. Oishi, N.; Iwata, H.; Kobayashi, N.; Fujimoto, K.; Yamaura, K. A survey on awareness of the "finger-tip unit" and medication guidance for the use of topical steroids among community pharmacists. *Drug Discov. Ther.* **2019**, *13*, 128–132. [CrossRef] [PubMed]
48. Teixeira, A.; Teixeira, M.; Herdeiro, M.T.; Vasconcelos, V.; Correia, R.; Bahia, M.F.; Almeida, I.F.; Vidal, D.G.; Sousa, H.F.P.E.; Dinis, M.A.P. Knowledge and practices of community pharmacists in topical dermatological treatments. *Int. J. Environ. Res. Public Health* **2021**, *18*, 2928. [CrossRef]
49. Raffin, D.; Giraudeau, B.; Samimi, M.; Machet, L.; Pourrat, X.; Maruani, A. Corticosteroid phobia among pharmacists regarding atopic dermatitis in children: A national French survey. *Acta Derm. Venereol.* **2016**, *96*, 177–180. [CrossRef] [PubMed]
50. Salzmann, S.; Salzmann, M.; Staubach, P. Compounded preparations in dermatology-analysis of prescribing habits in everyday clinical practice in Germany. *J. Dtsch. Dermatol. Ges.* **2020**, *18*, 334–340. [CrossRef]
51. Lambrechts, L.; Gilissen, L.; Morren, M.-A. Topical Corticosteroid Phobia Among Healthcare Professionals Using the TOPICOP Score. *Acta Derm. Venereol.* **2019**, *99*, 1004–1008. [CrossRef]
52. Giua, C.; Floris, N.P.; Schlich, M.; Keber, E.; Gelmetti, C. Dermatitis in community pharmacies: A survey on italian pharmacists' management and implications on corticophobia. *Pharmacia* **2021**, *68*, 671–677. [CrossRef]
53. Jairoun, A.A.; Al-Hemyari, S.S.; El-Dahiyat, F.; Shahwan, M. GAP analysis of pharmacy curriculum regarding topical corticosteroid use and safety. *J Public Health* **2021**, *29*, 1291–1299. [CrossRef]
54. Issa, A.Y.; Farhaa, R.A.; Elayeha, E.; Bustanji, Y. Impact of medical specialty on the prescription patterns of topical corticosteroid among healthcare professionals. *Jordan J. Pharm. Sci.* **2016**, *9*, 103–114. [CrossRef]
55. Thandar, Y.; Botha, J.; Mosam, A. Community pharmacists' knowledge, attitude and practices towards the use of complementary and alternative medicines in Durban, South Africa. *Health SA Gesondheid* **2019**, *24*, 6. [CrossRef] [PubMed]
56. Abed, A.S.; Hassan, J.K. Abuse of topical glucocorticoids among patients visiting community pharmacy in Basrah-Iraq. *Indian. J. Forensic Med. Toxicol.* **2021**, *15*, 623–632.

57. Balshem, H.; Helfand, M.; Schünemann, H.J.; Oxman, A.D.; Kunz, R.; Brozek, J.; Vist, G.E.; Falck-Ytter, Y.; Meerpohl, J.; Norris, S. GRADE guidelines: 3. Rating the quality of evidence. *J. Clin. Epidemiol.* **2011**, *64*, 401–406. [CrossRef]
58. Mays, N.; Pope, C.; Popay, J. Systematically reviewing qualitative and quantitative evidence to inform management and policy-making in the health field. *J. Health Serv. Res. Policy* **2005**, *10* (Suppl. S1), 6–20. [CrossRef] [PubMed]
59. Corticosteroïden: Niet dun smeren, maar per FTU. Koninklijke Nederlandse Maatschappij Pharmacie (KNMP). Available online: https://maken.wikiwijs.nl/userfiles/b/b0c1c845c5840e083a8a5fd7d1166c8ebeb71bdd.pdf (accessed on 16 November 2022).
60. Smith, S.D.; Hong, E.; Fearns, S.; Blaszczynski, A.; Fischer, G. Corticosteroid phobia and other confounders in the treatment of childhood atopic dermatitis explored using parent focus groups. *Australas. J. Dermatol.* **2010**, *51*, 168–174. [CrossRef]
61. Stalder, J.F.; Aubert, H.; Anthoine, E.; Futamura, M.; Marcoux, D.; Morren, M.A.; Trzeciak, M.; Szalai, Z.; Veres, K.; Deleuran, M. Topical corticosteroid phobia in atopic dermatitis: International feasibility study of the TOPICOP score. *Allergy* **2017**, *72*, 1713–1719. [CrossRef]
62. Nathan, A.D.; Shankar, P.R.; Sreeramareddy, C.T. Community pharmacists' counseling practices and patient experiences about topical corticosteroids–an online survey in the Klang Valley, Malaysia. *BMC Prim. Care* **2022**, *23*, 263. [CrossRef]
63. McMillan, S.S.; Thangarajah, T.; Anderson, C.; Kelly, F. Pharmacy student decision making in over-the-counter medicine supply: A critical incident study. *Res. Soc. Adm. Pharm.* **2018**, *14*, 749–757. [CrossRef]
64. Chahine, B.; Cherfane, M.; Sakr, F.; Safwan, J.; Dabbous, M.; Akel, M.; Rahal, M. Community pharmacists' perceptions and role in the management of common dermatological problems in Lebanon: A cross-sectional study. *Int. J. Pharm. Pract.* **2021**, *29*, 573–579. [CrossRef]
65. Garreau, A.C.; Stalder, J.F.; Méry, S.; Bunouf, P.; Jean-Decoster, C.; Nosbaum, A.; Eczema Foundation, t.F.G.o.T.E.i.D. Impact of an e-learning programme on pharmacists' management of atopic dermatitis. *J. Eur. Acad. Dermatol. Venereol.* **2021**, *35*, e656–e659. [CrossRef]
66. Fivenson, D. The effect of atopic dermatitis on total burden of illness and quality of life on adults and children in a large managed care organization. *J. Manag. Care Pharm.* **2002**, *8*, 333–342. [CrossRef] [PubMed]
67. Wollenberg, A.; Barbarot, S.; Bieber, T.; Christen-Zaech, S.; Deleuran, M.; Fink-Wagner, A.; Gieler, U.; Girolomoni, G.; Lau, S.; Muraro, A. Consensus-based European guidelines for treatment of atopic eczema (atopic dermatitis) in adults and children: Part I. *J. Eur. Acad. Dermatol. Venereol.* **2018**, *32*, 657–682. [CrossRef] [PubMed]
68. Wollenberg, A.; Kinberger, M.; Arents, B.; Aszodi, N.; Avila Valle, G.; Barbarot, S.; Bieber, T.; Brough, H.; Calzavara Pinton, P.; Christen-Zäch, S. European guideline (EuroGuiDerm) on atopic eczema–part II: Non-systemic treatments and treatment recommendations for special AE patient populations. *J. Eur. Acad. Dermatol. Venereol.* **2022**, *36*, 1904–1926. [CrossRef] [PubMed]

healthcare

MDPI

Article

Patient Safety Culture in the Southern Region of Saudi Arabia: A Survey among Community Pharmacies

Vigneshwaran Easwaran [1,*], Tahani Musleh Almeleebia [1], Mohammad Jaffar Sadiq Mantargi [2], Noohu Abdulla Khan [1], Sultan M. Alshahrani [1], Khalid Orayj [1], Osama Abdullh Amer Alshehri [1], Nawaf Yahya Hassan Alqasimi [1] and Saad A. AlFlan [1]

1 Department of Clinical Pharmacy, College of Pharmacy, King Khalid University, Abha 61421, Saudi Arabia
2 Department of Pharmacology, Batterjee Medical College, Jeddah 21442, Saudi Arabia; jaffar.sadiq@bmc.edu.sa
* Correspondence: vbagyalakshmi@kku.edu.sa

Abstract: Measuring patient safety culture in the community pharmacy can help with identifying areas for development. The current study is a descriptive, cross-sectional, electronic survey conducted among pharmacists working in community pharmacies located in the southern region of Saudi Arabia. The community pharmacy version of the "Pharmacy Survey on Patient Safety Culture" (PSOPSC) was used to collect data. The positive response rate (PRR) was calculated as per the guidance provided by the Agency for Healthcare Research and Quality (AHRQ). Based on the PRR, two least-achieved items (<25%) were taken for further analysis to identify the possible predictors. A sum of 195 pharmacists were included in this study and most of them were working in chain pharmacies. The highest PRRs were observed with teamwork (94.99), and patient counseling (94.13), followed by physical space and environment (93.07). The lowest PRRs were observed with staffing, work pressure, and pace (47.70), followed by communication openness (72.60). Specific characteristics, such as experience and the number of working hours, are significantly related to a poor PRR. The current study results indicate that the scope for improving patient safety exists in various areas of community pharmacies. However, it is necessary to prioritize the need based on a positive response rate.

Keywords: patient safety; positive response rate; community pharmacy

check for updates

Citation: Easwaran, V.; Almeleebia, T.M.; Mantargi, M.J.S.; Khan, N.A.; Alshahrani, S.M.; Orayj, K.; Alshehri, O.A.A.; Alqasimi, N.Y.H.; AlFlan, S.A. Patient Safety Culture in the Southern Region of Saudi Arabia: A Survey among Community Pharmacies. *Healthcare* **2023**, *11*, 1416. https://doi.org/10.3390/healthcare11101416

Academic Editor: Georges Adunlin

Received: 5 April 2023
Revised: 9 May 2023
Accepted: 10 May 2023
Published: 12 May 2023

1. Introduction

Patient safety is one of the critical pillars of healthcare systems around the world. Patient Safety is a healthcare discipline that emerged with the ongoing complexities of healthcare systems [1]. It has been reported by several researchers that pharmacy practice services can substantially improve patient safety and reduce hospital costs associated with medication errors [2,3].

The importance of patient safety is increasingly getting recognized worldwide nowadays [4]. A systemic review of patient safety culture in Arabic countries was performed and reported that it is important to promote the patient safety culture. Understanding the components and influencing factors of culture, and assessing the safety culture, is essential to developing strategies that create a culture committed to providing the safest possible care for patients [4,5]. The Kingdom of Saudi Arabia (KSA) has a well-established national-level medicine policy. This policy sets a direction for future development by focusing on institutional interconnection, improvement in cost-effective procurement and prescribing habits, a secure supply of good quality medicines, and the growth of the domestic pharmaceutical industry. It also establishes the patient's safety by tracking the medicines throughout the supply chain using an electronic track-and-trace system [6]. In Saudi Arabia, community pharmacies are still product oriented. In 2018, the Ministry of Health (MoH) in Saudi Arabia regulated and restricted the supply of antibiotics without prescription. In addition, MoH also launched an initiative to get medicines to the public from private community pharmacies free of charge, instead of taking them only from government hospitals. However, this raises a concern about patient safety in community pharmacies [7]. Most of the studies conducted in Arab countries utilized hospital surveys on patient safety culture (HSOPSC) [8,9]. However, easy accessibility and the quality of pharmacy practice services provided by community pharmacies make this setting a suitable place for disseminating patient safety. Thus, it is important to understand the real-life situation regarding various domains of patient safety culture in community pharmacies. Moreover, measuring patient safety culture can help with identifying areas for development and understanding the changes in practice over time [8]. Patient safety culture in health care is usually influenced by multiple factors within the healthcare organization and helps with the prevention and reduction of errors [10]. Therefore, understanding the patient safety culture of community pharmacies will be helpful to improving the quality of the KSA healthcare program, by raising pharmacists' awareness about patient safety issues and identifying areas of strengths as well as those that require improvement [11,12]. Numerous research studies are available in the context of patient safety from the perspective of various healthcare professionals, including pharmacists [13–15]. Despite the availability of abundant literature in this regard, there is still a scarcity of data concerning the assessment of patient safety culture in community pharmacy settings, particularly in the Kingdom of Saudi Arabia [16,17].

Hence, the current study was undertaken to analyze the patient safety culture and to identify the possible predictors and areas for improvement related to patient safety culture in community pharmacies located in the southern region of Saudi Arabia.

2. Materials and Methods

2.1. Study Design and Sampling

It was a descriptive, cross-sectional, survey-based study conducted among the pharmacists working in community pharmacies located in Abha, in the southern region of KSA. A non-probabilistic convenient sampling technique was used to recruit the study participants. All of the pharmacists working in community pharmacies located in this region were invited to participate in the survey, including student pharmacists, pharmacy technicians, and pharmacy assistants, even if more than one pharmacist was available in the same pharmacy.

2.2. Study Tool

The community pharmacy version of the "Pharmacy Survey on Patient Safety Culture" (PSOPSC) developed by the Agency for Healthcare Research and Quality (AHRQ) was used to collect data for the study [18]. It is a pre-validated, self-administered questionnaire that uses a 5-point Likert scale containing 40 items that measure 11 domains of patient safety culture. The domains included in the study are physical space and environment, teamwork, staff training and skills, communication openness, patient counseling, staffing work pressure and pace, communication about prescriptions across the shift, communication about mistakes, response to mistakes, organizational learning, continuous improvement, and overall perceptions.

2.3. Scoring and Positive Response Rate Calculation

The level of agreement for each item in the Likert scale ranged from strongly agree (5 points) to strongly disagree (1 point) for positively phrased items, and vice versa for negatively phrased items. The same condition was applied for a few items where the responses ranged from always (5 points) to never (1 point). The high scores (4 & 5) were perceived as positive responses and the scores of 1 and 2 were perceived as negative responses. The neutral response, missed response, and don't know responses were excluded for positive response ratio calculation. The level of agreement for each item in the Likert scale ranged from 5 points to 1 point. The scores of 1 & 2 were perceived as negative responses. The positive response rate was calculated according to the guidelines provided in the PSOPSC by the AHRQ. The calculation procedure is to divide the frequency of (scores of 4 & 5) positive responses by the total number of responses, with the exclusion of neutral and don't know responses.

Based on the positive response rate (PRR), the two least-achieved items were taken for further analysis to identify the possible sociodemographic predictors. The reliability was ensured by calculating the internal consistency using Cronbach's alpha for the whole questionnaire and individual domains, and it was found to be good.

2.4. Data Collection

Both the English and Arabic languages were used in the questionnaire to conduct the survey. The research assistants met the pharmacists in person at their pharmacies at a time that was convenient for them. They were given an electronic device filled with a survey form (Google Forms), and responses were collected in the pharmacy itself.

2.5. Data and Analysis

Necessary statistical analyses were performed using the Statistical Package for social sciences (SPSS) version 22, for windows (IBM Corp., Armonk, NY, USA). The chi-square test was used to identify the predictors related to the items that received the least positive response rate. A p-value less than 0.05 was considered significant.

2.6. Ethical Considerations

The study procedure and protocol were approved by the ethical committee of King Khalid University. Ethical approval # is ECM#2020-1102. The informed consent form was included at the beginning of the electronic survey questionnaire and only those participants who gave informed consent were allowed further access to the questionnaire to participate in the study.

3. Results

A total of 206 pharmacists were invited to participate in the survey; 11 among them have disagreed to provide electronic consent to participate in the survey. A total of 195 pharmacists were included in this study and among them, the majority (80%) were working in chain pharmacies. Among those included in the study, 17.4% were pharmacy managers, 64.1% were pharmacists, 13.3% were student pharmacists and 5.1% were pharmacy technicians. Around 131 (67.2%) pharmacists were males. Of the pharmacists included in the current study, 63.1% completed their Bachelor of Pharmacy degree. Furthermore, 23.1% of pharmacists completed their PharmD degree. Only 4.6% have completed a Master's degree in pharmacy. More than 50% of the pharmacists had less than 5 years of experience and 26.2% have experience of 6–10 years. Additionally, 6.7% of pharmacists have an experience of 11–15 years. The lowest percentage (4.1%) of pharmacists have an experience of 16–20 years. A total of 6.7% of the pharmacists have experience of more than 20 years. Among the community pharmacists included in the current study, 34.9% were handling more than 250 prescriptions per week and the remaining were handling less than 250 prescriptions. More than half of the community pharmacists were working more than 40 h per week. One quarter of the community pharmacists were not familiar with their patients and around half of the population (53.8%) were somewhat familiar with their patients. Furthermore, 20.5% of the community pharmacists were extremely familiar with their patients (Table 1).

The positive response ratio was calculated for the individual items and derived for various dimensions of patient safety culture (Table 2). The highest PRRs were observed with teamwork (94.99), and patient counseling (94.13), followed by physical space and environment (93.07). The least PRRs were observed with staffing, work pressure, and pace (47.70), followed by communication openness (72.60). The PRR ranged from 47.70 to 95 across various patient safety dimensions.

Table 1. Sociodemographic characteristics.

Characteristics	Number of Responses	Percentage
Pharmacy type		
Chain	162	83.1
Independent	33	16.9
Pharmacist position		
Managing Pharmacist	34	17.4
Pharmacist	125	64.1
Technicians	10	5.1
Student Pharmacist	26	13.3
Gender		
Male	131	67.2
Female	64	32.8
Last degree in pharmacy		
Bachelor	123	63.1
PharmD	45	23.1
Master's	9	4.6
Others	18	9.2
Year of experience		
Less than 5 years	110	56.4
6–10 years	51	26.2
11–15 years	13	6.7
16–20 years	8	4.1
More than 20 years	13	6.7
Prescription volume per week		
Less than 250	127	65.1
More than 250	68	34.9
Familiarity with patients		
Unfamiliar	50	25.6
Somewhat familiar	105	53.8
Extremely Familiar	40	20.5
Working hours per week		
30–40	94	48.2
More than 40	101	51.8

Table 2. Positive Response Rate (PRR) to patient safety culture dimensions [18].

Dimensions	Number of Positive Responses (Score of 5 & 4)	Number of Negative Responses (Score of 2 & 1)	Total Responses (Excluding Neutral and Don't Know Responses)	PRR (PRR = Number of Positive Responses/Total Responses × 100)
Physical space and environment				93.07
A1. This pharmacy is well organized	164	8	172	95.35
A5. This pharmacy is free of clutter/untidiness	153	11	167	91.62
A7. The physical layout of this pharmacy supports good workflow	143	12	155	92.26
Team work				94.99
A2. The staff treat each other with respect	166	10	176	94.32
A4. Staff in this pharmacy clearly understand their roles & responsibilities	162	9	171	94.74
A9. Staff work together as an effective team	164	7	171	95.91

Table 2. *Cont.*

Dimensions	Number of Positive Responses (Score of 5 & 4)	Number of Negative Responses (Score of 2 & 1)	Total Responses (Excluding Neutral and Don't Know Responses)	PRR (PRR = Number of Positive Responses/Total Responses × 100)
Staff training and skills				88.60
A3. Pharmacy assistants/helpers in this pharmacy receive the training they need to do their jobs	138	17	155	89.03
A6. Staff in this pharmacy have the skills they need to do their jobs well	151	14	165	91.52
A8. Staff who are new to this pharmacy receive adequate orientation	142	23	165	86.06
A10. Staff get enough training from this pharmacy	144	20	164	87.80
Communication openness				85.08
B1. Staff ideas and suggestions are valued in this pharmacy	119	35	154	77.27
B5. Staff feel comfortable asking questions when they are unsure about something	141	14	155	90.97
B10. It is easy for staff to speak up to their pharmacy manager (chief pharmacist) or pharmacy owner about patient safety concerns in this pharmacy	134	20	154	87.01
Patient counseling				94.13
B2. Pharmacists in this pharmacy encourage patients to talk about their medications	168	7	175	96.00
B7. Our pharmacists spend enough time talking to patients about how to use their medications	151	11	162	93.21
B11. Our pharmacists tell patients important information about their new prescriptions	150	11	161	93.17
Staffing, work pressure, and pace				47.70
B3. Staff take adequate breaks during their shifts	109	38	147	74.15
B9. We feel rushed when processing prescriptions	22	128	150	14.67
B12. We have enough staff to handle the workload	130	27	157	82.80
B16. Interruptions/distractions in this pharmacy (from phone calls, faxes, customers, etc.) make it difficult for staff to work accurately	29	122	151	19.21
Communication about prescriptions across shifts				86.84
B4. We have clear expectations about exchanging important prescription information across shifts	131	15	146	89.73
B6. We have standard procedures for communicating prescription information across shifts	134	26	160	83.75
B14. The status of problematic prescriptions is well communicated across shifts	141	21	162	87.04
Communication about mistakes				90.03
B8. Staff in this pharmacy discuss mistakes	132	19	151	87.42
B13. When patient safety issues occur in this pharmacy, staff discuss them	136	15	151	90.07
B15. In this pharmacy, we talk about ways to prevent mistakes from happening again	150	12	162	92.59
Responses to mistakes				73.82
C1. Staff are treated fairly when they make mistakes	155	10	165	93.94
C4. This pharmacy helps staff learn from their mistakes rather than punishing them	124	21	145	85.52
C7. We look at staff actions and the way we do things to understand why mistakes happen in this pharmacy	131	18	149	87.92
C8. Staff feel like their mistakes are held against them	43	111	154	27.92

Table 2. *Cont.*

Dimensions	Number of Positive Responses (Score of 5 & 4)	Number of Negative Responses (Score of 2 & 1)	Total Responses (Excluding Neutral and Don't Know Responses)	PRR (PRR = Number of Positive Responses/Total Responses × 100)
Organizational learning—continuous improvement				90.94
C2. When a mistake happens, we try to figure out what problems in the work process led to the mistake	153	10	163	93.87
C5. When the same mistake keeps happening, we change the way we do things	135	17	152	88.82
C10. Mistakes have led to positive changes in this pharmacy	137	15	152	90.13
Overall perceptions of patient safety				72.60
C3. This pharmacy places more emphasis on sales than on patient safety	63	94	157	40.13
C6. This pharmacy is good at preventing mistakes	133	15	148	89.86
C9. The way we do things in this pharmacy reflects a strong focus on patient safety	144	20	164	87.80

Considering the individual questions, the highest PRR was observed with B2 (Pharmacists in this pharmacy encourage patients to talk about their medications, 96), followed by A9 (Staff works together as an effective team, 95.91), and A1 (This pharmacy is well organized, 94.99).

The lowest PRR was observed with B9 (We feel rushed when processing prescriptions, 14.67), and B16 (Interruptions/distractions in this pharmacy make it difficult for staff to work accurately, 19.21) These two items contributed heavily to poor patient safety culture. Hence, these two dimensions were further analyzed to estimate the involvement of any sociodemographic predictors.

The results revealed that some specific demographic characteristics are significantly associated with the poor positive response rate. The year of experience is significantly associated with the PRR of the pace of processing prescriptions ($p = 0.023$). Working hours is another predictor involved in affecting patient safety by modifying the item known as "we feel rushed when processing prescriptions" ($p = 0.003$). None of the other sociodemographic characters are significantly associated with the item "B9" (we feel rushed when processing prescriptions) (Table 3).

Table 3. Predictors of the lowest scored item (B9) under the dimension of Staffing, work pressure, and pace.

Characteristics	Number of Positive Responses	Number of other Responses	*p*-Values
Pharmacy type			
Chain	20	142	0.298
Independent	2	31	
Pharmacist position			
Managing Pharmacist	2	32	0.730
Pharmacist	16	109	
Technicians	1	9	
Student Pharmacist	3	23	
Gender			
Male	16	115	0.556
Female	6	58	

Table 3. *Cont.*

Characteristics	Number of Positive Responses	Number of other Responses	*p*-Values
Last degree in pharmacy			
Bachelor	14	109	1.000
PharmD	5	40	
Master's	1	8	
Others	2	16	
Year of experience			
Less than 5 years	13	97	0.023 *
6–10 years	7	43	
11–15 years	1	10	
16–20 years	0	8	
More than 20 years	1	12	
Prescription volume per week			
Less than 250	12	115	0.269
More than 250	10	58	
Familiarity with patients			
Unfamiliar	2	48	0.162
Somewhat familiar	14	91	
Extremely Familiar	6	34	
Working hours per week			
30–40	18	76	0.003 *
More than 40	4	97	

Chi square test, * <0.05 considered significant.

The analysis of item B16 (Interruptions/distractions in this pharmacy make it difficult for staff to work accurately) shows that the type of pharmacy (p = 0.019) and the year of experience of pharmacists (0.003) are significantly impacting patient safety. Other sociodemographic characteristics are not showing any statistical significance (Table 4).

Table 4. Predictors of lowest scored item (B16) under the dimension of Staffing, work pressure, and pace.

Characteristics	Number of Positive Responses	Number of other Responses	*p*-Values
Pharmacy type			
Chain	22	140	0.019 *
Independent	7	26	
Pharmacist position			
Managing Pharmacist	6	28	0.511
Pharmacist	20	105	
Technicians	0	10	
Student Pharmacist	3	23	
Gender			
Male	15	116	0.550
Female	14	50	

Table 4. *Cont.*

Characteristics	Number of Positive Responses	Number of other Responses	p-Values
Last degree in pharmacy			
Bachelor	18	105	0.588
PharmD	8	37	
Master's	0	9	
Others	3	15	
Year of experience			
Less than 5 years	13	97	0.003 *
6–10 years	7	44	
11–15 years	6	7	
16–20 years	3	5	
More than 20 years	0	13	
Prescription volume per week			
Less than 250	20	107	0.638
More than 250	9	59	
Familiarity with patients			
Unfamiliar	7	43	0.304
Somewhat familiar	13	92	
Extremely Familiar	9	31	
Working hours per week			
30–40	14	80	1.000
More than 40	15	86	

Chi square test, * <0.05 considered significant.

Table 5 depicts the overall ratings with regard to the patient safety grade reported by the community pharmacies included in the study. It was observed that 49.7% & 29.7% of community pharmacies rated their pharmacy as excellent and very good, respectively. Additionally, 25% rated their pharmacy a lower patient safety grade. Only 25% of the community pharmacists reported positively that the overall patient safety grade is good or very good, or excellent.

Table 5. Overall patient safety grade in community pharmacy.

Overall Patient Safety Grade	Frequency	Percentage
Poor	1	5
Very good	8	4.1
Good	31	15.9
Very good	58	29.7
Excellent	97	49.7

4. Discussion

Most of the studies conducted in the past concerning patient safety culture focused on hospital settings. Very few studies have reported on community pharmacies. Our literature survey revealed that very few studies were conducted to report the trend of patient safety culture among community pharmacies in the Kingdom of Saudi Arabia.

Medication errors are the most frequent cause of a degraded patient safety culture in community pharmacies, according to research studies conducted all over the world [19,20]. However, it is equally important to identify the other possible reasons which may diminish patient safety. Therefore, it is essential to understand the concept of patient safety culture from the perspective of community pharmacists [1].

Using the PSOPSC, the current study investigated the patient safety culture from the community pharmacists' perspectives. The response rate of the current study was 92.8%, which shows community pharmacists' commitment to enhance patient safety; this percentage was found to be greater than that of prior studies in the field [3,21,22].

According to a study from Kuwait, the highest PRRs were observed for cooperation, organizational learning-continuous improvement, and patient counseling. These findings resemble our study almost exactly, where we found that teamwork and patient counseling had the highest PRRs [1].

The 36 elements of the questionnaire were added up to produce an overall mean score for patient safety, i.e., 82.32, which is similar to the Kuwait study (83.3) but higher than the studies from Malaysia and China [3,23]. The overall score about patient safety in the current study demonstrates that the community pharmacists from the southern part of Saudi Arabia are very well-aware of their responsibilities to improve patient safety. Teamwork showed the highest favorable response rate in our study. These findings are close to those of a study carried out among hospital pharmacists from Kuwait [24].

Similar findings were observed in hospital-based studies from Taiwan, Belgium, and the United States [25,26]. In addition to hospital pharmacists, studies conducted amongst community pharmacists also yielded a similar result to the current study [23,27].

Heavy workloads and inadequate staff contribute to mistakes in the pharmacy, which might lead to clinically significant problems [28,29]. In addition to our study, numerous domestic and international studies observed a lower PRR in staffing and work pressure. These findings suggest that pharmacists around the world feel the same way—that they do not have enough people to handle the workload, which has a direct impact on patient safety [1,3,21,23,26,30].

Communication openness among the pharmacy staff members within the pharmacy can help to prevent mistakes and improve patient safety [3]. Despite a higher PRR in communication openness, the mistakes were apparent. A lower PRR was observed in the domain "responses to mistake", specifically in the item "Staff feel like their mistakes are held against them". The staff members who committed mistakes usually had a variety of emotional distresses. Additionally, these results are in line with the study conducted in the United States [31]. The supportive culture within the work environment and constructive feedback may help those people to learn from mistakes [32].

The current study results indicated a positive approach by community pharmacists towards providing patient counseling and spending more time with the patients to explain the appropriate usage of medications. It was recommended by the World Health Organization that pharmacists must spend at least 3 min with the patients to provide patient counseling and orientation [33] and this tends to impact the patient outcome directly [34]. It is not surprising that the community pharmacists from our study showed a positive, and best, approach towards patient counseling because the role of the community pharmacist in patient counseling and appropriate patient counseling skills are taught in almost every pharmacy school in Saudi Arabia [35–37].

The study from central Saudi Arabia reported that the risk of dispensing error is continuously increasing [38], and the work environment is considered one of the great influencing factors of pharmacists' work [16]. Pharmacy errors are associated with the lack of adequate space and unfavorable environment. The current study indicated that most of the community pharmacies in the study region were well organized, free from clutter, and supported by a good workflow. These results are reflective of various national and international studies [3,5,23,30].

Most of the community pharmacists included in the current study satisfactorily rated their pharmacy on patient safety. However, the PRR was lower in one of the items included in this domain, which demonstrates that a few pharmacies were emphasizing sales more than patient safety. A study from Malaysia reported comparable results to our study [23]. The overall grade given by the pharmacists on patient safety was excellent, which is in line with a similar study published by Alsaleh FM et al. [1]. The current study attempted to figure out the possible predictor for the lowest-scored items. The pharmacists working in standalone pharmacies, highly experienced pharmacists, and pharmacists with high familiarity with patients were processing the prescriptions hastily during peak hours. The pharmacists who were working in independent pharmacies and who have high experience felt that they had frequent interruptions in their pharmacy, which made it difficult to work accurately.

Limitations

With a non-probabilistic convenient sampling method, the current study lacks generalizability; there might be the possibility for under or over-representation of the population. The current study is a self-reported questionnaire-based study that could be possibly influenced by response bias and socially desirable bias. Questionnaires are often completed voluntarily, leading to the risk of response bias, where only those who have had positive experiences may complete the questionnaire. This may interfere with the results and may provide a false impression regarding the patient safety culture in pharmacy practice and medicine. In addition, it is possible that respondents may provide answers that they feel are socially desirable, rather than truthful or reflective of their actual experiences. This can lead to distorted findings and inaccuracy in the results.

5. Conclusions

Pharmacists in the community must ensure medication safety throughout the medication use process. A strong culture of patient safety can help in appropriate utilization of resources. The current study shall provide basic evidence to design an appropriate future intervention and to direct available resources. Our study findings indicated that there was an overall positive perception among the community pharmacists in Abha concerning patient safety culture. It also pinpointed the strong points and potential areas that could use more development to enhance the culture of patient safety in neighborhood pharmacies. It reveals that the scope for improving patient safety exists among all of the domains. However, it is necessary to prioritize the need based on a positive response rate, preferably for the domain called staffing, work pressure, and pace. In addition, it is not a one-point end, but rather it requires continuous evaluation and monitoring to understand the change of practice due to time.

Author Contributions: Conceptualization, V.E. and T.M.A.; methodology, M.J.S.M. and N.A.K.; formal analysis, V.E., S.M.A. and K.O.; data curation, O.A.A.A., N.Y.H.A. and S.A.A.; writing—original draft preparation, V.E.; writing—review and editing, V.E. and N.A.K. All authors have read and agreed to the published version of the manuscript.

Funding: This research received no external funding.

Institutional Review Board Statement: The study was conducted in accordance with the Declaration of Helsinki, and approved by the ethical committee of King Khalid University. Ethical approval # ECM#2020-1102.

Informed Consent Statement: Electronic informed consent was obtained from all the community pharmacists involved in the study.

Data Availability Statement: Data from this study are available upon request from the corresponding author.

Acknowledgments: We acknowledge all the study participants.

Conflicts of Interest: The authors declare no conflict of interest.

References

1. Alsaleh, F.M.; Abahussain, E.A.; Altabaa, H.H.; Al-Bazzaz, M.F.; Almandil, N.B. Assessment of Patient Safety Culture: A Nationwide Survey of Community Pharmacists in Kuwait. *BMC Health Serv. Res.* **2018**, *18*, 884. [CrossRef] [PubMed]
2. Bond, C.A.; Raehl, C.L.; Franke, T. Clinical Pharmacy Services, Hospital Pharmacy Staffing, and Medication Errors in United States Hospitals. *Pharmacotherapy* **2002**, *22*, 134–147. [CrossRef] [PubMed]

3. Jia, P.L.; Zhang, L.H.; Zhang, M.M.; Zhang, L.L.; Zhang, C.; Qin, S.F.; Li, X.L.; Liu, K.X. Safety Culture in a Pharmacy Setting Using a Pharmacy Survey on Patient Safety Culture: A Cross-Sectional Study in China. *BMJ Open* **2014**, *4*, e004904. [CrossRef] [PubMed]
4. Elmontsri, M.; Almashrafi, A.; Banarsee, R.; Majeed, A. Status of Patient Safety Culture in Arab Countries: A Systematic Review. *BMJ Open* **2017**, *7*, e013487. [CrossRef]
5. Aljaffary, A.; Al Yaqoub, F.; Al Madani, R.; Aldossary, H.; Alumran, A. Patient Safety Culture in a Teaching Hospital in Eastern Province of Saudi Arabia: Assessment and Opportunities for Improvement. *Risk Manag. Healthc. Policy* **2021**, *14*, 3783–3795. [CrossRef]
6. Almoteiry, K.; Alharf, A.; Al Hammad, B.; Aljuffali, I.; Al-Azemi, N.; Al-Ghaith, T.; Alhomidi, S.; Alshehri, A.; Seiter, A.; Herbst, C.; et al. National Medicines Policy Development, Saudi Arabia. *Bull. World Health Organ.* **2022**, *100*, 511–519. [CrossRef]
7. Al Juffali, L.A.; Knapp, P.; Al-Aqeel, S.; Watson, M.C. Medication Safety Problems Priorities in Community Pharmacy in Saudi Arabia: A Multi-Stakeholder Delphi Study Using the Human Factors Framework. *BMJ Open* **2019**, *9*, e032419. [CrossRef]
8. Alswat, K.; Abdalla, R.A.M.; Titi, M.A.; Bakash, M.; Mehmood, F.; Zubairi, B.; Jamal, D.; El-Jardali, F. Improving Patient Safety Culture in Saudi Arabia (2012–2015): Trending, Improvement and Benchmarking. *BMC Health Serv. Res.* **2017**, *17*, 516. [CrossRef]
9. Alrasheedy, A.A.; Hassali, M.A.; Wong, Z.Y.; Aljadhey, H.; AL-Tamimi, S.K.; Saleem, F. Pharmaceutical Policy in Saudi Arabia. In *Pharmaceutical Policy in Countries with Developing Healthcare Systems*; Babar, Z.-U.-D., Ed.; Springer International Publishing: Cham, Switzerland, 2017; pp. 329–347, ISBN 978-3-319-51673-8.
10. Joint Commision; Joint Commision International. WHO Collaborating Center for Patient Safety's Nine Life-Saving Patient Safety Solutions. *Jt. Comm. J. Qual. Patient Saf.* **2007**, *33*, 427–462.
11. Rasheed, M.K.; Alqasoumi, A.; Hasan, S.S.; Babar, Z.-U.-D. The Community Pharmacy Practice Change towards Patient-Centered Care in Saudi Arabia: A Qualitative Perspective. *J. Pharm. Policy Pract.* **2020**, *13*, 59. [CrossRef]
12. Al-jedai, A.; Qaisi, S.; Al-meman, A. Pharmacy Practice and the Health Care System in Saudi Arabia. *Can. J. Hosp. Pharm.* **2016**, *69*, 231–237. [CrossRef] [PubMed]
13. El-Jardali, F.; Sheikh, F.; Garcia, N.A.; Jamal, D.; Abdo, A. Patient Safety Culture in a Large Teaching Hospital in Riyadh: Baseline Assessment, Comparative Analysis and Opportunities for Improvement. *BMC Health Serv. Res.* **2014**, *14*, 122. [CrossRef] [PubMed]
14. Hamdan, M.; Saleem, A.A. Assessment of Patient Safety Culture in Palestinian Public Hospitals. *Int. J. Qual. Health Care* **2013**, *25*, 167–175. [CrossRef] [PubMed]
15. Khater, W.A.; Akhu-Zaheya, L.M.; Al-Mahasneh, S.I.; Khater, R. Nurses' Perceptions of Patient Safety Culture in Jordanian Hospitals. *Int. Nurs. Rev.* **2015**, *62*, 82–91. [CrossRef] [PubMed]
16. Phipps, D.L.; Noyce, P.R.; Parker, D.; Ashcroft, D.M. Medication Safety in Community Pharmacy: A Qualitative Study of the Sociotechnical Context. *BMC Health Serv. Res.* **2009**, *9*, 158. [CrossRef]
17. Lawati, M.H.A.L.; Dennis, S.; Short, S.D.; Abdulhadi, N.N. Patient Safety and Safety Culture in Primary Health Care: A Systematic Review. *BMC Fam. Pract.* **2018**, *19*, 104. [CrossRef]
18. Internet Citation: Community Pharmacy Survey on Patient Safety Culture. Content Last Reviewed March 2023; Agency for Healthcare Research and Quality: Rockville, MD, USA. Available online: https://www.ahrq.gov/sops/surveys/pharmacy/index.html (accessed on 1 April 2023).
19. Odukoya, O.K.; Stone, J.A.; Chui, M.A. E-Prescribing Errors in Community Pharmacies: Exploring Consequences and Contributing Factors. *Int. J. Med. Inform.* **2014**, *83*, 427–437. [CrossRef]
20. Ashcroft, D.M.; Quinlan, P.; Blenkinsopp, A. Prospective Study of the Incidence, Nature and Causes of Dispensing Errors in Community Pharmacies. *Pharmacoepidemiol. Drug. Saf.* **2005**, *14*, 327–332. [CrossRef]
21. Ali, H.; Ibrahem, S.Z.; Al Mudaf, B.; Al Fadalah, T.; Jamal, D.; El-Jardali, F. Baseline Assessment of Patient Safety Culture in Public Hospitals in Kuwait. *BMC Health Serv. Res.* **2018**, *18*, 158. [CrossRef]
22. Herner, S.J.; Rawlings, J.E.; Swartzendruber, K.; Delate, T. Pharmacy Survey on Patient Safety Culture: Benchmarking Results. *J. Patient Saf.* **2017**, *13*, 37–42. [CrossRef]
23. Sivanandy, P.; Maharajan, M.K.; Rajiah, K.; Wei, T.T.; Loon, T.W.; Yee, L.C. Evaluation of Patient Safety Culture among Malaysian Retail Pharmacists: Results of a Self-Reported Survey. *Patient Prefer. Adherence* **2016**, *10*, 1317–1325. [CrossRef] [PubMed]
24. Badr, H.E.; AlFadalah, T.; El-Jardali, F. Towards Promoting Patient Safety Practices: Baseline Assessment of Patient Safety Culture in Three Private Hospitals. *Int. J. Healthc. Manag.* **2020**, *13*, 207–214. [CrossRef]
25. Smits, M.; Christiaans-Dingelhoff, I.; Wagner, C.; van der Wal, G.; Groenewegen, P.P. The Psychometric Properties of the "Hospital Survey on Patient Safety Culture" in Dutch Hospitals. *BMC Health Serv. Res.* **2008**, *8*, 230. [CrossRef] [PubMed]
26. Hellings, J.; Schrooten, W.; Klazinga, N.; Vleugels, A. Challenging Patient Safety Culture: Survey Results. *Int. J. Health Care Qual. Assur.* **2007**, *20*, 620–632. [CrossRef] [PubMed]
27. Jayasingam, S.; Ansari, M.A.; Jantan, M. Influencing Knowledge Workers: The Power of Top Management. *Ind. Manag. Data Syst.* **2010**, *110*, 134–151. [CrossRef]
28. James, K.L.; Barlow, D.; Bithell, A.; Hiom, S.; Lord, S.; Pollard, M.; Roberts, D.; Way, C.; Whittlesea, C. The Impact of Automation on Workload and Dispensing Errors in a Hospital Pharmacy. *Int. J. Pharm. Pract.* **2013**, *21*, 92–104. [CrossRef]

29. Malone, D.C.; Abarca, J.; Skrepnek, G.H.; Murphy, J.E.; Armstrong, E.P.; Grizzle, A.J.; Rehfeld, R.A.; Woosley, R.L. Pharmacist Workload and Pharmacy Characteristics Associated with the Dispensing of Potentially Clinically Important Drug-Drug Interactions. *Med. Care* **2007**, *45*, 456–462. [CrossRef]
30. Almalki, Z.S.; Alshehri, A.M.; Alturki, L.A.; Altamimi, R.A.; Albassam, A.A.; Alqurashi, M.S.; Saleh Al-Omaim, F.A.; Ahmed, N. Exploring Patient-Safety Culture in the Community Pharmacy Setting: A National Cross-Sectional Study. *Postgrad. Med.* **2021**, *133*, 57–65. [CrossRef]
31. Aboneh, E.A.; Stone, J.A.; Lester, C.A.; Chui, M.A. Evaluation of Patient Safety Culture in Community Pharmacies. *J. Patient Saf.* **2020**, *16*, e18–e24. [CrossRef]
32. Kroll, L.; Singleton, A.; Collier, J.; Rees Jones, I. Learning Not to Take It Seriously: Junior Doctors' Accounts of Error. *Med. Educ.* **2008**, *42*, 982–990. [CrossRef]
33. Al Qarni, H.; Alrahbini, T.; AlQarni, A.M.; Alqarni, A. Community Pharmacist Counselling Practices in the Bisha Health Directorate, Saudi Arabia -Simulated Patient Visits. *BMC Health Serv. Res.* **2020**, *20*, 745. [CrossRef] [PubMed]
34. Okumura, L.M.; Rotta, I.; Correr, C.J. Assessment of Pharmacist-Led Patient Counseling in Randomized Controlled Trials: A Systematic Review. *Int. J. Clin. Pharm.* **2014**, *36*, 882–891. [CrossRef] [PubMed]
35. Bawazeer, G.; Sales, I.; Alsunaidi, A.; Aljahili, S.; Aljawadi, M.H.; Almalag, H.M.; Alkofide, H.; Adam Mahmoud, M.; Alayoubi, F.; Aljohani, M. Student-Led Discharge Counseling Program for High-Risk Medications in a Teaching Hospital in Saudi Arabia: A Pilot Study. *Saudi Pharm. J.* **2021**, *29*, 1129–1136. [CrossRef] [PubMed]
36. Fathelrahman, A.I.; Alrobaian, M.; Altowayan, W.M.; Maghrabi, I.; Asiri, Y.A. Pharmacy Education in Saudi Arabia: Achievements and Challenges during the Last Two Decades with a Focus on Taif University as a Case Study. *Saudi Pharm. J.* **2022**, *30*, 649–654. [CrossRef] [PubMed]
37. Alshahrani, S.M.; Khan, N.A.; Easwaran, V.; Iqbal, M.J.; Alavudeen, S.S. Effects of Virtual Education on Clinical Pharmacy Practice in Saudi Arabia: Implementation of Simulation-Based Education. *Lat. Am. J. Pharm.* **2020**, *39*, 2520–2526.
38. Al-Arifi, M.N. Community Pharmacists' Attitudes toward Dispensing Errors at Community Pharmacy Setting in Central Saudi Arabia. *Saudi Pharm. J.* **2014**, *22*, 195–202. [CrossRef]

healthcare

MDPI

Article

Community Pharmacists' Perceptions of Their Role in Provision of Anemia Management in Jazan Region, Saudi Arabia, and the Associated Barriers

Osama A. Madkhali [1,*] and **Fahad Alzahrani** [2]

1 Department of Pharmaceutics, College of Pharmacy, Jazan University, Jazan 45124, Saudi Arabia
2 Clinical and Hospital Pharmacy Department, College of Pharmacy, Taibah University, Madinah 42353, Saudi Arabia; fzahrani@taibahu.edu.sa
* Correspondence: omadkhali@jazanu.edu.sa

Abstract: Background: As a result of the lack of research exploring community pharmacists' perspectives on anemia care, this study examined the perceived practices and barriers to anemia management services in Saudi Arabia. Methods: A questionnaire was administered to community pharmacists to validate pharmacist perceptions of their role in anemia care. Using an 11-item role test, pharmacists were asked about their perceptions of anemia management. Pharmacy anemia management barriers were explored using 20 items, and their perceptions of inter-professional contact were examined by two items. Data analyses were performed using SPSS version 22. Results: This research involved 324 community pharmacists, 62.3% of whom were males. There were significant differences between the location of pharmacy education and the perceived practice of anemia management. The most common barriers to anemia counseling were patients' lack of knowledge about anemia, health beliefs, patients' perceptions that their doctor takes care of them, and time constraints. The majority of respondents said they would like to have more contact with other healthcare professionals regarding the care of anemia patients. Conclusions: A positive perception of pharmacists' role in anemia management is prevalent among Saudi pharmacists in the Jazan region. Anemia management is challenging due to time limitations and patient-related problems.

Keywords: anemia management; perceived practice; barriers; community pharmacy; perceptions

Citation: Madkhali, O.A.; Alzahrani, F. Community Pharmacists' Perceptions of Their Role in Provision of Anemia Management in Jazan Region, Saudi Arabia, and the Associated Barriers. *Healthcare* **2022**, *10*, 1452. https://doi.org/10.3390/healthcare10081452

Academic Editors: Georges Adunlin and Eiji Nakatani

Received: 8 June 2022
Accepted: 29 July 2022
Published: 2 August 2022

1. Introduction

Anemia is a blood illness marked by a lack of healthy red blood cells capable of transporting enough oxygen to the tissues [1]. It affects a large number of people around the world, especially in developing countries, resulting in a huge financial burden due to the high cost of medical care [2]. The World Health Organization (WHO) has revealed that anemia affects nearly a quarter of the world's population, particularly newborns and women [3]. The prevalence of anemia in the Middle East (25 to 35%) is comparable to that in underdeveloped nations [1,5], in contrast to 5–8% prevalence in developed countries.

It has been reported that anemia is prevalent in 30–56% of Saudi Arabians [6]. Due to factors such as consanguineous marriages among first-degree families, lack of effective screening programs, and malaria epidemics, the Jazan region in the southern region of Saudi Arabia is one of the areas most affected by a group of inherited red blood cell disorders, particularly sickle cell anemia (SCA) [4]. Anemia is characterized by symptoms such as severe pain, acute chest syndrome, cerebrovascular accidents, recurring infections, hypoxia, and growth impairment [7]. These symptoms necessitate timely treatment and cooperation from all health specialists, including pharmacists.

Several studies have shown the role of healthcare specialists in the management of many chronic diseases [8–12]. Pharmacists have demonstrated a good impact on the management of different diseases such as diabetes [13], hypertension [14], and asthma [15].

Since anemia is a symptom-related disease, anemia management is very significant for either the patients themselves or the healthcare specialists. Early detection and treatment of the symptoms help in reducing the risk of morbidity and mortality, eliminating the complications of anemia, including frequent hospitalizations or allogeneic blood transfusion, and reducing cost [16–19]. Therefore, the role of healthcare community is to improve the quality of life of anemic patients by creating a shared quality improvement program that helps in all aspects of anemia management. Community pharmacists have significant participation in anemia management due to the frequent visit of anemic patients to the pharmacy.

In recent years, the scope of the practice of community pharmacists has increased appreciably to include the provision of services aimed at improving health outcomes [20]. Arising from their expertise in drugs, constant interaction with patients, and easy accessibility, pharmacists are in a unique position to assist patients in managing chronic illnesses [7,20,21]. Ironically, pharmacists are frequently underutilized in the provision of improved anemia management in primary care [22]. Community pharmacies represent the initial point of contact for many people who require healthcare in poor and underdeveloped nations [23]. Therefore, community pharmacists play a critical role in the treatment of chronic illnesses, an example of which is anemia.

To date, no research has been conducted to assess the perception of community pharmacists regarding their potential role in anemia management in the Jazan region of Saudi Arabia. As a result, the purpose of this study was to assess community pharmacists' perceptions of anemia management practices and barriers.

2. Materials and Methods

2.1. Study Design and Eligibility Criteria

From October to December 2020, a descriptive cross-sectional study was conducted among community pharmacists in the Jazan region of Saudi Arabia. All full licensed Saudi Arabian pharmacists working in community pharmacies in the Jazan region with a bachelor's degree or higher were eligible to participate in this study. In 2017, approximately 600 pharmacists practiced in the Jazan region of Saudi Arabia [24]. Using Raosfot®'s online sample size calculator, it was estimated that the minimum effective sample size in this study was 234, with a 95% confidence interval and a 5% error margin.

2.2. Sampling Procedure

Community pharmacists were recruited using convenience sampling. Six trained research assistants presented the study design and objectives to the community pharmacists. A link to the questionnaire was given to pharmacists who agreed to participate in the study, and they were asked to complete the questionnaire while the research assistants were on duty. Using this method, any issues raised during data collection were addressed consistently so as to enhance the degree of response. For pharmacists who were not seen during the first visit due to other engagements, the research assistants were asked to schedule another appointment at their convenience so that the study could be continued at a later date.

2.3. Data Collection

The responses were collected using a structured, self-administered questionnaire. The questionnaire used for this study was developed and modified based on the literature review [25–30] and the experience of the investigators (Table 1). The self-administered questionnaire comprised four sections. In the first section (demographics), the community pharmacists were required to provide information on nine demographic questions: age, gender, level of education, place where pharmacy degree was obtained, number of years of practice as licensed pharmacists in Saudi Arabia, degree of interest of pharmacists in anemia management, history of attendance/participation in structured or organized continuing education programs on anemia management, and estimates of the number of anemia patients they interacted with each week.

Table 1. The 33-item community pharmacist's role in anemia management questionnaire.

Section 1 (Role): The Pharmacists' Perception of Their Role Towards Anemia Management
Please indicate your level of agreement on each of the following statements about the role of a pharmacist when dealing with an anemic patient: 1. Conduct a drug history, including prescription medications, OTC, Herbal, and natural products 2. Describe the appropriate time to administer oral iron supplements 3. Describe potential adverse effects of iron supplements 4. Assist with food-food and food-drug interaction 5. Assist with the selection of more efficient supplements 6. Provide basic information on diet as it relates to anemia management 7. Provide basic information on exercise as it relates to anemia management 8. Counsel on medications that can exacerbate conditions 9. Counsel on signs and symptoms of anemia 10. Anemia self-management by the patient (i.e., recognizing when and knowing how to take action when anemia gets worse) 11. Refer patients who need to seek medical attention
Section 2 (Barrier): Barriers that Prevent Pharmacists from Providing Anemia Healthcare
Please indicate to what extent you feel each of the following factors impacts the pharmacist's ability to provide specific anemia counseling or services: 1. Lack of time by the pharmacist 2. Lack of time by the patient 3. Pharmacists' perception that it is not their role 4. Patient's perception that it is not the pharmacist's role 5. Language barriers 6. Patient's health beliefs 7. Patient's lack of anemia knowledge 8. Patient perception that they are already well cared for by the doctor 9. Conflict between professional and commercial interests 10. Trying not to 'overstep' the role of the doctor 11. No financial incentive 12. Difficulty to know patient's needs 13. Lack of counseling space 14. Lack of governmental or employer support
Lack of Confidence or skills in:
15. Anemia medication counseling 16. Anemia adherence counseling 17. Anemia self-management counseling 18. Anemia trigger factor counseling 19. Reviewing and counseling about anemia control 20. Anemia monitoring
Section 3 (Inter-professional contact):
Please indicate your level of agreement with each of the following statements: 1. I have good interprofessional contact with other healthcare professionals with regard to care of my patients with anemia 2. I would like to have more contact with other healthcare professionals with regards to the care of my patients with anemia

In the second part of the survey (role), 11 questions were posed to the community pharmacists who responded on a five-point Likert scale ranging from 1 (strongly disagree) to 5 (strongly agree). Each item was rated 4 or 5, depending on how well it was received.

In the third section (barriers), there were 20 barriers that militated against the provision of pharmacy anemia management services. A five-point Likert scale was used to assess how these barriers influenced the ability of community pharmacists to provide specific anemia counseling or services. The score on the five-point Likert scale ranged from 1 (no impact) to 5 (high impact). The last section of the questionnaire was based on inter-professional contact, and responses were ranked on a five-point Likert scale (1 = strongly disagree, 5 = strongly agree).

Two faculty members in the College of Pharmacy at Jazan University evaluated and reviewed the validity of the questionnaire items. The survey items were rated according to their relevance on a scale of 1–5, with 1 indicating that the item was not relevant, and 5 indicated that the item was highly relevant. The reviewers decided a priori to include in the final questionnaire only those statements rated as pertinent or highly relevant. Disputes in ratings between the two reviewers were resolved through discussion and compromise. A pilot test ($n = 7$) was used to evaluate the clarity and comprehension of the items included in the questionnaire. Pilot group comments and feedback led to minor changes in the study tool. These changes were intended to enhance the clarity of the survey items. The pilot sample data were excluded from the final analysis. Cronbach's alpha (an index of reliability) was evaluated for internal consistency. A Cronbach's alpha of more than 70% was taken as indicative of internal consistency [31].

2.4. Statistical Analysis

The data obtained in this study were analyzed using the IBM Statistical Package for the Social Sciences (SPSS Inc., Chicago, IL, USA) version 22. Data were analyzed using descriptive statistics such as percentages, means, and standard deviations. The Shapiro–Wilk tests were used to assess scores for normality of distribution. In the absence of normal distribution, the Mann–Whitney test and Kruskal–Wallis test were used. Values of $p = 0.05$ were considered indicative of statistically significant differences. All p values were two-sided.

2.5. Ethical Approval

Approval for this study was received from the Human Research Ethics Committee of Taibah University in Madinah, Saudi Arabia (COPTU-REC-22; 24 September 2021). All pharmacists involved in this research signed informed consent prior to their enrollment.

3. Results

3.1. Internal Consistencies

The study questionnaire items were internally consistent, as indicated by an overall Cronbach's alpha value of 83.9%. Cronbach's alpha values were also computed separately for each of the domains in the study. The values of Cronbach's alpha for 11 roles and current practice, 20 barrier items, and 2 inter-professional contacts were 96.8, 92.6, and 50%, respectively.

3.2. Demographics

In this study, 324 out of 600 community pharmacists were recruited in the Jazan region, Saudi Arabia. This met the sample size requirement, and the resultant response was 54.6%. The ages of the community pharmacists ranged from 21 to 60 years, with a mean age of 29.53 years. The majority of participants (62.3%) were males, and most of them (75.5%) hold PharmD. More than half of the participants (56.8%) graduated from the University of Jazan. The average years of pharmacy practice (experience) ranged from 0 to 12, while the average years of experience as licensed pharmacists in Saudi Arabia ranged from 0 to 10. Almost half of them ($n = 268$) indicated an interest in counseling anemia patients, despite the fact that most pharmacists ($n = 204$) had never participated in continuing education programs related to anemia management. Table 2 shows other demographic and pharmacy practice characteristics.

Table 2. Demographic and practice characteristics.

Characteristics	n (%)
Age	
21–29	202 (62.3)
30–39	101 (31.2)
40–49	20 (6.2)
50–60	1 (.3)
Gender	
Male	201 (62.3)
Female	122 (37.7)
Years as a pharmacist	
0–2	146 (45.1)
3–5	90 (27.8)
6–10	64 (19.8)
>10	24 (7.4)
Years as a licensed pharmacist in Saudi Arabia	
0–2	156 (48.1)
3–5	94 (29.0)
6–10	60 (18.5)
>10	14 (4.3)
Level of Education	
BSc.	78 (24.1)
PharmD	244 (75.5)
MSc	2 (0.6)
Source of Education	
University of Jazan	184 (56.8)
Other Saudi Universities	55 (17)
Foreign University	85 (26.2)
Interesting in counseling Anemia	
Yes	268 (82.71)
No	56 (17.31)
Attendance of Continuing Education Events Related to Anemia Management	
Yes	204 (63.00)
No	120 (37.00)
Number of Patients with Anemia seen in a Typical Week	
0–5	234 (72.23)
6 to 10	61 (18.81)
11 to 20	18 (5.61)
More than 20	11 (3.4)

3.3. *Community Pharmacists' Perceptions of Their Role in Anemia Management*

More than half of the studied pharmacists (74.4%) believed that community pharmacists play an important role in counseling anemia patients. Approximately 21% of pharmacists ($n = 71$) strongly agreed that pharmacists should be interested in patient's drug history comprising prescriptions, OTC, herbal products, and natural products. Moreover, 24.1% of the pharmacists ($n = 78$) strongly agreed that pharmacists should explain to anemic patients the potential adverse effects of iron supplements. The majority of the pharmacists (20.4%; $n = 66$) strongly agreed that anemic patients should receive counseling on medications that may worsen anemic conditions, while 71 pharmacists (20.4%) strongly agreed on counseling on signs and symptoms of anemia. However, 92 pharmacists (28.4%) were neutral on self-management of anemia. There was almost a unanimous agreement among 29.3% of the pharmacists that part of their role was to refer patients who required medical attention to their pharmacies. The detailed responses of the pharmacists are provided in Table 3.

Table 3. Perceived roles of pharmacists in counseling patients with anemia.

Item Number	Items	Strongly Disagree *n* (%)	Disagree *n* (%)	Neutral *n* (%)	Agree *n* (%)	Strongly Agree *n* (%)
1	Conduct a drug history, including prescription medications, OTC, Herbal, and natural products.	23 (7.1)	29 (9.0)	67 (20.7)	134 (41.4)	71 (21.9)
2	Describe the appropriate time to administer oral iron supplements.	22 (6.8)	27 (8.3)	71 (21.9)	128 (39.5)	76 (23.6)
3	Describe potential adverse effects of iron supplements.	26 (8.0)	28 (8.6)	62 (19.1)	130 (40.1)	78 (24.1)
4	Assist with drug-drug and food-drug interaction	21 (6.5)	28 (8.6)	77 (23.8)	115 (35.5)	83 (25.6)
5	Assist with the selection of more efficient supplements.	25 (7.7)	32 (9.9)	79 (24.4)	123 (38.0)	65 (20.1)
6	Provide basic information on diet as it relates to anemia management.	31 (9.6)	41 (12.7)	74 (22.8)	115 (35.5)	63 (19.3)
7	Provide basic information on exercise as it relates to anemia management.	25 (7.7)	50 (15.4)	88 (27.2)	109 (33.6)	52 (16.0)
8	Counsel on medications that can exacerbate conditions.	25 (7.7)	29 (9.0)	79 (24.4)	118 (36.4)	66 (20.4)
9	Counsel on signs and symptoms of anemia	27 (8.3)	29 (9.0)	79 (24.4)	118 (36.4)	71 (21.9)
10	Anemia self-management by the patient.	25 (7.7)	33 (10.2)	92 (28.4)	116 (35.8)	58 (17.9)
11	Refer patients who need to seek medical attention	27 (8.3)	32 (9.9)	61 (18.8)	109 (33.6)	95 (29.3)

The Kruskal–Wallis H test was applied to compare the mean differences in perceived practice scores among different groups with respect to age, level of education, the place from where their academic degree was obtained, number of years of practice as a pharmacist, number of years of practice as a licensed pharmacist in Saudi Arabia, and number of patients with anemia seen in a typical week. The Mann–Whitney U test was applied to compare mean differences in gender and attendance of continuing education events related to anemia management. These results are presented in Table 4. There was a significant relationship between pharmacy educational sources and perceptions of anemia management. Pharmacists who graduated from foreign universities had a more positive perception of their practice than pharmacists who graduated from Saudi universities. However, there was no significant relationship between respondents' age, gender, ethnicity, and duration of practice.

Table 4. Distribution of perceived practice of anemia according to socio-demographic variables.

Variables	Groups	*n*	Mean ± SD	*p*-Value
Age	21–29	202	3.46 ± 1.11	0.73
	30–39	101	3.71 ± 0.82	
	40–49	20	3.63 ± 0.85	
	50–60	1	3.00 ± -	
Gender	Male	201	3.61 ± 0.97	0.13
	Female	122	3.44 ± 1.06	
Years as a pharmacist	0–2	146	3.38 ± 1.10	0.10
	3–5	90	3.74 ± 0.91	
	6–10	64	3.72 ± 0.82	
	>10	24	3.31 ± 1.11	

Table 4. *Cont.*

Variables	Groups	*n*	Mean ± SD	*p*-Value
Years as a licensed pharmacist in SA	0–2	156	3.43 ± 1.10	0.45
	3–5	94	3.71 ± 0.90	
	6–10	60	3.54 ± 0.98	
	>10	14	3.67 ± 0.79	
Level of education	BSc.	78	3.75 ± 089	0.12
	PharmD	244	3.48 ± 1.01	
	MSc	2	3.36 ± 0.77	
Source of education	University of Jazan	184	3.47 ± 1.09	0.04
	Other Saudi Universities	55	3.35 ± 0.97	
	Foreign University	85	3.83 ± 0.76	
Interesting in counseling anemia	Yes	268	3.57 ± 1.01	0.20
	No	56	3.41 ± 1.00	
Attendance of continuing education events related to anemia management	Yes	204	3.61 ± 103	0.32
	No	120	3.43 ± 0.96	
No. of patients with anemia seen in a typical week	0–5	234		
	6–10	61		
	11–20	18		
	>20	11		

More than half of the participants indicated that each of the 20 potential barriers had some impact. The pharmacists identified the four most common barriers which impacted their ability to provide anemia services. These comprised a lack of awareness of anemia by patients, health beliefs of patients, patients' confidence in the care being provided by their doctors, and time constraints on the part of the patients. In terms of patient-related factors, language barriers and the patient's perception of the pharmacist's role were two factors that posed the greatest obstacles. In contrast, the pharmacists indicated that lack of financial incentive and conflict between professional and commercial interests did not have significant impacts on their ability to provide specific anemia services. The barriers identified as potential obstacles to anemia management by community pharmacists are shown in Tables 5 and 6.

Table 5. Perceived practice barriers to pharmacist's ability to provide specific anemia counseling or service.

Item Number	Item	No Impact *n* (%)	Slight Impact *n* (%)	Moderate Impact *n* (%)	Considerable Impact *n* (%)	High Impact *n* (%)
1	Lack of time by the pharmacist	41 (12.7)	42 (13.0)	123 (38.0)	71 (21.9)	47 (14.5)
2	Lack of time by the patient	32 (9.9)	51 (15.7)	104 (32.1)	52 (16.0)	85 (26.2)
3	Pharmacists' perception that it is not their role.	47 (14.5)	56 (17.3)	110 (34.0)	38 (11.7)	73 (22.5)
4	Patient's perception that it is not the pharmacist's role	43 (13.3)	50 (15.4)	111 (34.3)	71 (21.9)	49 (15.1)
5	Language barriers	86 (26.5)	55 (17.0)	85 (26.2)	66 (20.4)	32 (9.9)
6	Patient's health beliefs	29 (9.0)	56 (17.3)	113 (34.9)	75 (23.1)	51 (15.7)
7	Patient's lack of anemia knowledge	25 (7.7)	44 (13.6)	121 (37.3)	67 (20.7)	67 (20.7
8	Patient perception that they are already well cared for by the doctor	30 (9.3)	38 (11.7)	103 (31.8)	82 (25.3)	71 (21.9)
9	The conflict between professional and commercial interests	51 (15.7)	57 (17.6)	115 (35.5)	63 (19.4)	38 (11.7)
10	Trying not to 'overstep' the role of the doctor	38 (11.7)	62 (19.1)	115 (35.5)	75 (23.1)	34 (10.5)
11	No financial incentive	56 (17.3)	63 (19.4)	109 (33.6)	63 (19.4)	33 (10.2)
12	Difficulty to know patient's needs	42 (13.0)	57 (17.6)	110 (34.0)	80 (24.7)	35 (10.8)
13	Lack of counseling space	47 (14.5)	51 (15.7)	99 (30.6)	83 (25.6)	44 (13.6)
14	Lack of governmental or employer support	62 (19.1)	45 (13.9)	96 (29.6)	70 (21.6)	51 (15.7)

Table 6. Lack of confidence or skills.

Item Number	Items	No Impact *n* (%)	Slight Impact *n* (%)	Moderate Impact *n* (%)	Considerable Impact *n* (%)	High Impact *n* (%)
1	Anemia medication counseling	72 (22.2)	87 (26.9)	81 (25.0)	64 (19.8)	20 (6.2)
2	Anemia adherence counseling	62 (19.1)	93 (28.7)	91 (28.1)	59 (18.2)	19 (5.9)
3	Anemia self-management counseling	62 (19.1)	94 (29.0)	85 (26.2)	65 (20.1)	18 (5.6)
4	Anemia trigger factor counseling	54 (16.7)	79 (24.4)	107 (33.0)	66 (20.4)	18 (5.6)
5	Reviewing and counseling about anemia control	61 (18.8)	79 (24.4)	98 (30.2)	65 (20.1)	21 (6.5)
6	Anemia monitoring	59 (18.2)	83 (25.6)	90 (27.8)	67 (20.7)	25 (7.7)

3.4. Community Pharmacists' Perceived Level of Inter-Professional Contact

Approximately 36.1% of community pharmacists stated that they had good inter-professional contact when caring for patients with anemia, while 57.1% of the pharmacists said they would like to have more inter-professional contacts. Details of these responses are shown in Table 7.

Table 7. Inter-professional contact.

Item Number	Item	Strongly Disagree *n* (%)	Disagree *n* (%)	Neutral *n* (%)	Agree *n* (%)	Strongly Agree *n* (%)
1	I have good interprofessional contact with other healthcare professionals with regard to the care of my patients with anemia.	55 (17.0)	57 (17.36)	95 (29.3)	83 (25.6)	34 (10.5)
2	I would like to have more contact with other healthcare professionals with regard to the care of my patients with anemia.	23 (7.1)	30 (9.3)	84 (25.9)	89 (27.5)	96 (29.6)

4. Discussion

With a score of 70.8 ± 1.1, it is evident that community pharmacists had a positive perception of their role in anemia care. Pharmacists perceived that their role in anemia management involved three major components: patient self-management, medication use, and anemia control. This is consistent with extant literature showing positive perceptions regarding the role of community pharmacists in the management of chronic diseases [32–34]. Furthermore, our results indicated that the guidelines for managing anemic patients did not stipulate the role of a typical community pharmacist in Jazan, Saudi Arabia. Thus, the perception of community pharmacists about their role might be of prime importance in the future management of anemia.

More than half of the community pharmacists believed that they should provide advice to patients on how to monitor, control, and manage anemia. It is important for patients to understand the timing of administration of oral iron supplements, as well as the potential adverse effects of iron supplements and medications which may exacerbate anemia. On average, 58% of the pharmacists (n = 188) perceived the need to assist patients with selecting effective and efficient supplements.

A significant number of community pharmacists (198; 61%) counseled patients on drug–drug interactions, while 54.8% of the pharmacists (n = 178) gave advice on diets in connection with anemia management. However, only 161 of the community pharmacists (49.6%) indicated that they counseled patients on exercise in connection with anemia management. Similar findings were reported in previous studies [25,27].

This study observed a significant difference between pharmacy educational sources and perceived anemia management practices. Those pharmacists who graduated from foreign universities had a more positive perception of their practice than those who graduated from Saudi universities. A possible explanation for this result is that most pharmacy schools' curriculums in Saudi Arabia do not prepare graduates well enough to provide chronic disease management services, including anemia. Alaqeel and Abanmy found that many Saudi pharmacy schools do not offer any training in a community pharmacy before graduation [35]. In addition, pharmacy interns are currently limited to filling prescriptions in a community pharmacy without anything to do with counseling or providing other services [36].

The study found that both community pharmacists and anemic patients encountered significant and common barriers to anemia counseling. In terms of factors related to community pharmacists, 35% or more indicated that the most significant barriers to anemia counseling were insufficient time, difficulty in knowing patients' needs, lack of counseling space, and the lack of government or employer support. Patients' lack of time, the perception that it is not the role of pharmacists to treat anemia, health beliefs, lack of knowledge about anemia, and the patient's confidence in the care being provided by doctors, were the most prominent barriers related to anemia counseling. Similar types of barriers were identified in previous studies [25,27,37]. Furthermore, 204 (63%) of the community pharmacists expressed interest in participating in continuing education programs related to anemia management. In order to improve anemia management and enhance health care outcomes in the future, it is necessary to develop an anemia educational care program to enhance pharmacists' knowledge and awareness about anemia and also provide patient counseling points for pharmacists to consider when discussing anemia [38].

Moreover, this study investigated the expectations of pharmacists regarding their interprofessional relationships in light of the fact that international and national guidelines for anemia management advocate a multidisciplinary approach. In spite of the fact that most participants had contact with other health care professionals regarding the care of anemic patients, almost 57% of the pharmacists would like to have more of these interactions. It is clear from existing literature that inter-professional relationships are critical to anemia management [27]. Although the current study did not investigate this issue further, the strength of the responses to this question, and the identification of strong barriers militating against the perceived roles of physicians and pharmacists, suggest the need for more studies in this area.

This study has several strengths, such as a high response rate from recruited respondents and internal consistency in responses, as measured by Cronbach's alpha. However, the study has some limitations. In the first place, it was conducted only among pharmacists in one region of Saudi Arabia (Jazan). Thus, the findings of this study cannot be applied to the entire population of community pharmacists in Saudi Arabia. Secondly, since the study was cross-sectional, the findings obtained are only correlational, not causal. Lastly, the questionnaire was developed based on current anemia management guidelines, previous research, and expert opinion, without qualitative research.

5. Conclusions

The pharmacists had a positive perspective on improved management of anemia. Patients were perceived to have a three-dimensional role in anemia care; these comprised self-management, medication use, and anemia control. Furthermore, this study has identified barriers to anemia counseling from the perspective of both pharmacists and patients. There were several barriers to providing anemia services, such as time and patient concerns. Research should be conducted in the future to determine barriers to the expansion of community pharmacists' roles in anemia management, given the current international push to manage chronic diseases in primary care and the evidence that pharmacy-based disease state management services could benefit patients.

Author Contributions: Conceptualization: O.A.M. and F.A.; methodology: F.A.; software: F.A.; validation: O.A.M. and F.A.; formal analysis: F.A.; investigation: O.A.M.; resources: O.A.M.; data curation: O.A.M.; writing (original draft preparation): F.A.; writing (review and editing): O.A.M.; visualization: O.A.M.; supervision: O.A.M.; project administration: O.A.M. All authors have read and agreed to the published version of the manuscript.

Funding: The authors extend their appreciation to the Deputyship for Research and Innovation, Ministry of Education in Saudi Arabia, for funding this research work through project number RUP20-01.

Institutional Review Board Statement: The study was approved by the Research ethics committee of the College of Pharmacy, Taibah University, Madinah. Saudi Arabia (COPTU-REC-22; 24 September 2021)

Informed Consent Statement: Not applicable.

Data Availability Statement: Data are available upon reasonable request by contacting the corresponding author.

Conflicts of Interest: The authors declare no conflict of interest.

References

1. Walker, H.K.; Hall, W.D.; Hurst, J.W. *Clinical Methods: The History, Physical, and Laboratory Examinations*; Butterworths: Oxford, UK, 1990.
2. Turner, J.; Parsi, M.; Badireddy, M. *Anemia*; StatPearls Publishing: Treasure Island, FL, USA, 2022.
3. McLean, E.; Cogswell, M.; Egli, I.; Wojdyla, D.; De Benoist, B. Worldwide prevalence of anaemia, WHO vitamin and mineral nutrition information system, 1993–2005. *Public Health Nutr.* **2009**, *12*, 444–454. [CrossRef] [PubMed]
4. Piel, F.B.; Hay, S.I.; Gupta, S.; Weatherall, D.J.; Williams, T.N. Global burden of sickle cell anaemia in children under five, 2010–2050: Modelling based on demographics, excess mortality, and interventions. *PLoS Med.* **2013**, *10*, e1001484. [CrossRef] [PubMed]
5. Stoltzfus, R.J. Iron deficiency: Global prevalence and consequences. *Food Nutr. Bull.* **2003**, *24*, S99–S103. [CrossRef] [PubMed]
6. Verster, A.; Vander Pols, J.C. *Anaemia in the Eastern Mediterranean Region*; World Health Organization: Geneva, Switzerland, 1995.
7. Ogunfowora, O.B.; Olanrewaju, D.M.; Akenzua, G.I. A comparative study of academic achievement of children with sickle cell anemia and their healthy siblings. *J. Natl. Med. Assoc.* **2005**, *97*, 405. [PubMed]
8. Allegrante, J.P.; Wells, M.T.; Peterson, J.C. Interventions to support behavioral self-management of chronic diseases. *Annu. Rev. Public Health* **2019**, *40*, 127. [CrossRef]
9. Pasquel, F.J.; Lansang, M.C.; Dhatariya, K.; Umpierrez, G.E. Management of diabetes and hyperglycaemia in the hospital. *Lancet Diabetes Endocrinol.* **2021**, *9*, 174–188. [CrossRef]
10. Al Sulayyim, H.J.; Al Omari, A.; Badri, M. An assessment for diagnostic and therapeutic modalities for management of pediatric Iron defficiency Anemia in Saudi Arabia: A crossectional study. *BMC Pediatr.* **2019**, *19*, 314. [CrossRef] [PubMed]
11. Al Zahrani, S.; Eid Alosaimi, M.; Alamrim, A.; Alotaibi, M.; Almatar, E.A.; Almanea, B.A. Association between knowledge and drug adherence in patients with hypertension in Saudi Arabia. *Arch. Pharma. Pract.* **2019**, *10*, 71–76.
12. Hamdan, A.-J.; Wali, S.; Salem, G.; Al-Hameed, F.; Almotair, A.; Zeitouni, M.; Aref, H.; Nadama, R.; Algethami, M.M.; Al Ghamdy, A. Asthma control and predictive factors among adults in Saudi Arabia: Results from the Epidemiological Study on the Management of Asthma in Asthmatic Middle East Adult Population study. *Ann. Thorac. Med.* **2019**, *14*, 148.
13. Almanasef, M.; Almaghaslah, D.; Kandasamy, G.; Vasudevan, R.; Batool, S. Involvement of community pharmacists in public health services in Asir Region, Saudi Arabia: A cross-sectional study. *Int. J. Clin. Pract.* **2021**, *75*, e14940. [CrossRef]
14. Almansour, H.A.; Aloudah, N.M.; Alhawassi, T.M.; Chaar, B.; Krass, I.; Saini, B. Health consumer engagement in developing novel preventive health community pharmacy roles in cardiovascular disease in Saudi Arabia: A qualitative analysis. *Saudi Pharm. J.* **2020**, *28*, 529–537. [CrossRef] [PubMed]
15. Said, A.S.; Hussain, N.; Kharaba, Z.; Al Haddad, A.H.; Abdelaty, L.N.; Roshdy, R.R. Knowledge, attitude, and practice of pharmacists regarding asthma management: A cross-sectional study in Egypt. *J. Pharm. Policy Pract.* **2022**, *15*, 35. [CrossRef] [PubMed]
16. Shander, A.; Goodnough, L.T.; Javidroozi, M.; Auerbach, M.; Carson, J.; Ershler, W.B.; Ghiglione, M.; Glaspy, J.; Lew, I. Iron deficiency anemia—Bridging the knowledge and practice gap. *Transfus. Med. Rev.* **2014**, *28*, 156–166. [CrossRef] [PubMed]
17. Shander, A.; Javidroozi, M.; Ozawa, S.; Hare, G. What is really dangerous: Anaemia or transfusion? *Br. J. Anaesth.* **2011**, *107*, i41–i59. [CrossRef] [PubMed]
18. Zilinski, J.; Zillmann, R.; Becker, I.; Benzing, T.; Schulz, R.-J.; Roehrig, G. Prevalence of anemia among elderly inpatients and its association with multidimensional loss of function. *Ann. Hematolo.* **2014**, *93*, 1645–1654. [CrossRef]
19. Goodnough, L.T.; Maniatis, A.; Earnshaw, P.; Benoni, G.; Beris, P.; Bisbe, E.; Fergusson, D.; Gombotz, H.; Habler, O.; Monk, T. Detection, evaluation, and management of preoperative anaemia in the elective orthopaedic surgical patient: NATA guidelines. *Br. J. Anaesth.* **2011**, *106*, 13–22. [CrossRef] [PubMed]
20. Kelly, D.V.; Young, S.; Phillips, L.; Clark, D. Patient attitudes regarding the role of the pharmacist and interest in expanded pharmacist services. *Can. Pharm. J.* **2014**, *147*, 239–247. [CrossRef]
21. Bailey, J.E.; Surbhi, S.; Bell, P.C.; Jones, A.M.; Rashed, S.; Ugwueke, M.O. SafeMed: Using pharmacy technicians in a novel role as community health workers to improve transitions of care. *J. Am. Pharm. Assoc.* **2016**, *56*, 73–81. [CrossRef]
22. Watkins, K.; Fisher, C.; Misaghian, J.; Schneider, C.R.; Clifford, R. A qualitative evaluation of the implementation of guidelines and a support tool for asthma management in primary care. *Asthma Res. Pract.* **2016**, *2*, 8. [CrossRef] [PubMed]

23. Khanal, S.; Nissen, L.; Veerman, L.; Hollingworth, S. Pharmacy workforce to prevent and manage non-communicable diseases in developing nations: The case of Nepal. *Res. Soc. Adm. Pharm.* **2016**, *12*, 655–659. [CrossRef] [PubMed]
24. AlRuthia, Y.; Alsenaidy, M.A.; Alrabiah, H.K.; AlMuhaisen, A.; Alshehri, M. The status of licensed pharmacy workforce in Saudi Arabia: A 2030 economic vision perspective. *Hum. Resour. Health* **2018**, *16*, 28. [CrossRef]
25. Akram, W.; Ijaz, N.; Ahmad, H.; Jamshaid, M.; Ismail, N.E. Barriers to the provision of asthma services and perceived practice towards asthma management among urban community pharmacists in Selangor, Malaysia. *Braz. J. Pharm. Sci.* **2019**, *54*, e17324. [CrossRef]
26. Debenito, J.M.; Billups, S.J.; Tran, T.S.; Price, L.C. Impact of a clinical pharmacy anemia management service on adherence to monitoring guidelines, clinical outcomes, and medication utilization. *J. Manag. Care Pharm.* **2014**, *20*, 715–720. [CrossRef] [PubMed]
27. Kritikos, V.S.; Reddel, H.K.; Bosnic-Anticevich, S.Z. Pharmacists' perceptions of their role in asthma management and barriers to the provision of asthma services. *Int. J. Pharm. Pract.* **2010**, *18*, 209–216. [CrossRef]
28. Kucera, A.; Smith, B.; Tsu, L.V. Anemia and the Role of the Pharmacist. *Ariz. J. Pharm.* **2014**, 31–35.
29. Saibaba, S.V.; Ramu, B. Role of Community Pharmacist in Management of Anaemia. *Clin. Med.* **2018**, *6*, 5–9.
30. Weil, E.; Oxencis, C. Pharmacist collaborative practice agreement for the management of anemia in malignant disease with erythropoiesis-stimulating agents. *Support. Care Cancer* **2015**, *23*, 2507–2513. [CrossRef]
31. Thigpen, N.N.; Kappenman, E.S.; Keil, A. Assessing the internal consistency of the event-related potential: An example analysis. *J. Psychophysiolo.* **2017**, *54*, 123–138. [CrossRef]
32. Verma, R.K.; Chong, W.W.; Taha, N.A.; Paraidathathu, T. A Qualitative Study Exploring Community Pharmacists' Experiences and Views About Weight Management Interventions and Services in Klang Valley, Malaysia. *Front. Public Health* **2021**, *9*, 1288. [CrossRef]
33. Al Haqan, A.A.; Al-Taweel, D.M.; Awad, A.; Wake, D.J. Pharmacists' attitudes and role in diabetes management in Kuwait. *Med. Princ. Pract.* **2017**, *26*, 273–279. [CrossRef]
34. Mukattash, T.L.; Jarab, A.S.; Mukattash, I.; Nusair, M.B.; Farha, R.A.; Bisharat, M.; Basheti, I.A. Pharmacists' perception of their role during COVID-19: A qualitative content analysis of posts on Facebook pharmacy groups in Jordan. *Pharm. Pract.* **2020**, *18*, 1900. [CrossRef] [PubMed]
35. Alaqeel, S.; Abanmy, N.O. Counselling practices in community pharmacies in Riyadh, Saudi Arabia: A cross-sectional study. *BMC Health Serv. Res.* **2015**, *15*, 557. [CrossRef] [PubMed]
36. Al-Arifi, M.N. Patients' perception, views and satisfaction with pharmacists' role as health care provider in community pharmacy setting at Riyadh, Saudi Arabia. *Saudi Pharm. J.* **2012**, *20*, 323–330. [CrossRef] [PubMed]
37. Loh, P.; Chua, S.S.; Karuppannan, M. The extent and barriers in providing pharmaceutical care services by community pharmacists in Malaysia: A cross-sectional study. *BMC Health Serv. Res.* **2021**, *21*, 822. [CrossRef]
38. Hedima, E.W.; Adeyemi, M.S.; Ikunaiye, N.Y. Community pharmacists: On the frontline of health service against COVID-19 in LMICs. *Res. Soc. Adm. Pharm.* **2021**, *17*, 1964–1966. [CrossRef]

healthcare

MDPI

Article

Community Pharmacists' Experiences and Attitudes towards the Provision of Sexual and Reproductive Health Services: An International Survey

Javiera Navarrete [1], Christine A. Hughes [1,*], Nese Yuksel [1], Theresa J. Schindel [1], Shigeo Yamamura [2], Tomoko Terajima [3], Tatta Sriboonruang [4], Chanthawat Patikorn [4] and Puree Anantachoti [4]

1 Faculty of Pharmacy and Pharmaceutical Sciences, College of Health Sciences, University of Alberta, Edmonton, AB T6G 2H1, Canada
2 Faculty of Pharmaceutical Sciences, Josai International University, Chiba 283-8555, Japan
3 Faculty of Pharmaceutical Sciences, Shonan University of Medical Sciences, Kanagawa 244-0806, Japan
4 Faculty of Pharmaceutical Sciences, Chulalongkorn University, Bangkok 10330, Thailand
* Correspondence: christine.hughes@ualberta.ca; Tel.: +1-780-492-5903

Abstract: Access to comprehensive sexual and reproductive health (SRH) services remains a challenge worldwide. Describing community pharmacists' SRH services in countries with different scopes of practice will aid in understanding how pharmacists view their roles and how to support them in providing needed services. A cross-sectional web-based survey was administered to pharmacists working in community pharmacies in Japan, Thailand, and Canada. The survey covered 7 SRH categories: pregnancy tests, ovulation tests, contraception, emergency contraception, sexually transmitted and blood-borne infections, maternal and perinatal health, and general sexual health. Descriptive statistics were used to analyze the data. A total of 922 eligible responses were included in the analysis (Japan = 534, Thailand = 85, and Canada = 303). Most Thai and Canadian participants reported dispensing hormonal contraceptives (Thailand = 99%, Canada = 98%) and emergency contraceptive pills (Thailand = 98%, Canada = 97%). Most Japanese participants provided patient education on barrier contraceptives for men (56%) and information on the safety of medications in pregnancy (74%) and breastfeeding (76%). The majority of participants expressed interest in additional training and expanding their roles in SRH. Sharing international experiences can guide challenges faced by the evolution of pharmacists' practice in SRH. Providing pharmacists support could help their readiness for this role.

Keywords: sexual health; reproductive health; pharmacists; community pharmacy services; survey; international cooperation

Citation: Navarrete, J.; Hughes, C.A.; Yuksel, N.; Schindel, T.J.; Yamamura, S.; Terajima, T.; Sriboonruang, T.; Patikorn, C.; Anantachoti, P. Community Pharmacists' Experiences and Attitudes towards the Provision of Sexual and Reproductive Health Services: An International Survey. *Healthcare* **2023**, *11*, 1530. https://doi.org/10.3390/healthcare11111530

Academic Editor: Georges Adunlin

Received: 24 April 2023
Revised: 19 May 2023
Accepted: 22 May 2023
Published: 24 May 2023

1. Introduction

Access to comprehensive sexual and reproductive health (SRH) services remains a challenge worldwide. According to the World Health Organization (WHO), 4.3 billion people of reproductive age worldwide will not have access to at least one SRH intervention in their lifetime [1]. More recently, the COVID-19 pandemic has significantly impacted the provision of these services [2–9]. Fear of accessing in-person care, medication shortage, suspended services and care programs have limited access to SRH services during the pandemic [2,3,8]. As the current global agenda includes ensuring accessible and high-quality SRH services for everyone [10], finding more options for access to these services is important.

The evolution of pharmacy practice is an international phenomenon. Development, adoption, and integration of new roles and responsibilities by pharmacists have been the trend over the past few decades [11–13]. Balancing professional, clinical and economic considerations and adopting new roles of pharmacists are challenges for the profession worldwide [14]. Evidence for the benefits of pharmacists' involvement in the delivery of

SRH services is growing. Pharmacists have been recognized as competent and trustworthy healthcare professionals expanding access to a wide range of SRH services [15,16]. A scoping review highlighted that pharmacists' roles in SRH have evolved beyond traditional product-focused services, such as treatment of sexually transmitted and bloodborne infections (STBBI) and contraception prescribing [16]. Challenges with the provision of SRH services by pharmacists reported in studies include integration into the pharmacy daily workflow, remuneration, cost and reimbursement for patients, and policy regulations [16]. However, most literature is from the US and UK, and there is little research describing international contexts and identifying how pharmacists can serve those needing to access SRH services.

Several factors prevent the translation of contemporary patient-oriented pharmacy practice models globally [17,18]. One of these factors is the quality and availability of information about pharmacists' current scope of practice [17,18]. Pharmacy practice has steadily advanced over the past few decades, but significant variations in the scope of practice have been described [19]. As there is a lack of universal practice standards across pharmacy settings and countries due to differences in healthcare systems, public health agenda, pharmacy curricula, professional regulations, continuing education, and pharmacists' compensation for professional services [18], research highlighting these differences is crucial to understand the current state of SRH services and opportunities to influence and promote further expansion of pharmacist' roles in this area [17,20].

Given the prominent role in communities as part of primary health care, describing community pharmacists' SRH services in countries with a different scope of practice will aid in understanding how pharmacists view their roles, see themselves as SRH providers, and what support they need to provide SRH services. To our knowledge, there is limited information regarding pharmacists' experiences as SRH providers in Canada [21–24], and no research has described SRH services in Thailand and Japan. This study aims to explore SRH services provided by pharmacists practicing in community pharmacies in Japan, Thailand, and Canada. The secondary objectives are to identify perceived factors influencing the delivery of services and training preferences to support role expansion in each country.

1.1. Study Context

Pharmacy Education and Scope of Practice

The general characteristics and differences among educational programs, pharmacy regulations, and scope of practice between Japan, Canada, and Thailand are highlighted in Table 1.

The number of years required to obtain a pharmacy degree is similar in these countries. In Japan, completing the extended Bachelor of Pharmacy (6 years) is mandatory to qualify for the national examination for entry to practice. Influenced by the US-Thai consortium, Thailand developed their first Doctor of Pharmacy (PharmD) program in 1999. Since 2014, a 6-year PharmD program has been compulsory for national licensure [25]. Pharmacy programs in Canada implemented the PharmD degree by 2020 [26].

The scope of practice differs in each country. In Canada, Alberta is the province with the broadest scope of practice and was the first to implement prescribing authority for pharmacists in 2007 [27]. Legislation in Alberta allows pharmacists to access information in patients' electronic health records, administer drugs by injection, order laboratory tests, and prescribe medications, including independent prescribing (additional prescribing authorization or APA) [27,28]. As a result, pharmacists in Alberta can prescribe hormonal contraception and administer progestin-only injectable contraceptives, as well as vaccines.

Pharmacy practice in Japan is principally focused on dispensing medications and providing patient counselling [29]. However, authorities and professionals in Japan are exploring how pharmacists' roles could address different health needs [29]. Sexual freedom, recognition of health risks, and access to SRH services are current public health concerns [30]. Pharmacists are ideally situated to enhance access to services. Currently, the scope of practice allows Japanese pharmacists to counsel and educate patients on SRH topics such as pregnancy and ovulation tests, contraception as well as dispense medications prescribed by a physician [30,31].

In the last decade, Thailand has expanded community pharmacists' roles to meet the needs of the public. After more than 10 years since transitioning to a 6-year PharmD program [32], community pharmacists offer medication reviews, risk assessments, smoking cessation and some screening services [33,34]. As part of the Universal Health Coverage Scheme, the community pharmacy is a primary care unit of the system, and pharmacists are involved in addressing several public health concerns, including adolescent pregnancy and birth rates, STBBI incidence and treatment rates [35–37].

Table 1. General characteristics, pharmacy education, and practice in Japan, Thailand, and Canada.

	Japan	Thailand	Canada
General characteristics [38–42]			
Population (millions)	125.7	71.6	38.25
Licensed pharmacists	302,500	47,525	48,134
Community Pharmacies	180,415	20,516	11,554
Pharmacy education [26,35,43–45]			
No. of pharmacy educational programs	74	19	10
Current academic credential	BPharm	PharmD	PharmD
Length of current program (years)	6	6	4
Pre-pharmacy requirements (years)	-	-	2
First year of transition from BPharm to a PharmD program (or extended BPharm)	2003	1999	2007
Completion year of transition to an all-PharmD (or extended BPharm) program	2006	2010	2020
National examination for entry to practice	Yes	Yes	Yes
Community pharmacy scope of practice [27–29,33,45–48]			
Availability of open-shelf drugs at the pharmacy	No	Yes	Yes
Dispensing prescription medications	Yes	Yes	Yes
Prescribing authorization	No	No	Yes
Administration of injections	No	No	Yes
Performing assessment based on symptoms	No	Yes	Yes
Performing point-of-care testing	No	No	Yes
Patient counselling and education	Yes	Yes	Yes

BPharm, Bachelor of Science in Pharmacy; PharmD, Doctor of Pharmacy.

2. Materials and Methods

2.1. Study Design

This was a descriptive, cross-sectional international study using survey methods. Results were analyzed and reported following the Strengthening the Reporting of Observational Studies in Epidemiology (STROBE) reporting guideline for cross-sectional studies [49].

An anonymous, web-based survey was distributed electronically in Japan, Thailand, and Canada (Alberta) using REDCap. REDCap is an electronic data capture tool hosted by the Women & Children's Health Research Institute at the University of Alberta [50,51]. The survey was directed to pharmacists working in a community setting. Initially, a screening question was used to capture this information and access the survey.

The survey was conducted from June 2020 to June 2021, with each country distributing the survey at different times. The period to collect responses was 1 to 6 months; in Thailand and Japan, the survey was open for 6 months due to slower response. Details about the strategies used are provided in Table 2.

Table 2. Procedures for data collection.

	Japan	Thailand	Canada
Recruitment strategy	Emails were sent to contact lists from pharmacy professional organizations, pharmacy and drugstore chains, and community pharmacist groups. Attendees of continuing education conferences. Facebook and Twitter promotion [52].	Emails sent to contact list from regional professional pharmacy associations	Emails sent to contact list from the regional professional regulatory body (Alberta)
Distribution	Email	Email	Email
Total number of pharmacists contacted	N/A	760 *	5349 *
Responses	534	85	303
Estimated response rate	N/A	N/A	8% [53]
Reminders	None	3	3
Dates of data collection	November 2020–April 2021	December 2020–June 2021	June 2020–July 2020
Duration of open survey	6 months	6 months	2 months
Incentive	None	None	$100 gift card draw (odds of winning 1 in 10)

* Total number of people contacted. This number includes pharmacists working in different settings, not only community pharmacy. N/A, not available.

2.2. Instrument

The development and content of the survey have been described previously [52,53]. The instrument was developed by the research team. A literature review informed the content, and the instrument was reviewed by experts in each country. The survey was first developed in English, then translated into Japanese and Thai, and adapted to each country's scope of pharmacist practice. The research team members and experts from Japan and Thailand reviewed the instrument for accurate translation.

The survey covered 7 common SRH categories: pregnancy tests, ovulation tests, contraception (non-hormonal and hormonal), emergency contraception, sexually and blood-borne transmitted infections, maternal and perinatal health, and general sexual health, and included 6 sections: demographics, provision of SRH services, attitudes towards the provision of SRH services, confidence when educating patients on SRH topics, factors influencing the provision of SRH services, and additional training preferences (Supplementary File S1). The survey distributed in Alberta covered additional topics reflecting the scope of practice in the region, such as the administration of injections and prescribing. Findings related to the expanded scope of practice in Alberta [53] and attitudes and practices of Japanese pharmacists regarding reproductive health services [52] have been previously published.

2.3. Variables

A 5-point Likert-type scale was used to assess attitudes towards (strongly disagree, disagree, neutral, agree, strongly agree) and factors influencing the provision of SRH services (no impact on the services, no effect on the services, little impact on the services, neutral, somewhat impacts the services, impacts the services to a great extent). The primary outcomes were the proportion of participants providing SRH services, the proportion of participants agreeing (or disagreeing) with a series of statements regarding pharmacists as SRH providers and the influence of factors in the provision of SRH services. Secondary outcomes were the proportion of participants interested in expanding their roles in SRH and additional training preferences, including SRH knowledge and competencies.

2.4. Bias

Survey responses were anonymous. A neutral language was used when designing the survey questions to minimize response bias. Increasing the number of days the survey was open and sending invitation and reminder emails were strategies used to reduce non-response bias and improve response rates [54–56].

2.5. Sample Size

There was no sample size set a priori.

2.6. Data Analysis

For analysis, eligibility was defined as submitted survey responses. Partial and unsubmitted responses were not included. Descriptive statistics were used to analyze the variables. Analysis was performed using Microsoft®Excel v.16.70 (Microsoft Corporation 2018).

2.7. Ethical Approval

This study received approval from the Josai International University Research Ethics Review Committee (10M200001), the Chulalongkorn University Research Ethics Review Committee (114.1/63), and the University of Alberta Health Research Ethics Board (Pro00095881).

3. Results

3.1. Participants

A total of 1,265 pharmacists attempted the survey (Japan = 743, Thailand = 121, Canada = 401), and 922 eligible responses from community pharmacists were included in the analysis (Japan = 534, Thailand = 85, Canada = 303). Participants were primarily female and between 20 and 40 years of age (Table 3). Regarding education and experience, most participants had a Bachelor of Pharmacy degree (Japan = 94%, Thailand = 55%, Canada = 79%). In Japan and Canada, most worked in a corporate/chain pharmacy (61% and 57%, respectively), whereas 79% worked in an independent pharmacy in Thailand.

Table 3. Participants characteristics.

Characteristics	**Japan (N = 534)** *n* **(%)**	**Thailand (N = 85)** *n* **(%)**	**Canada (N = 303)** *n* **(%)**
Gender			
Female	295 (55)	54 (64)	199 (66)
Age range			
20–30 years	208 (39)	17 (20)	71 (24)
31–40 years	116 (22)	40 (47)	120 (40)
41–50 years	97 (18)	11 (13)	60 (20)
51–60 years	81 (15)	8 (9)	41 (14)
61–70 years	29 (5)	7 (8)	9 (3)
71+ years	3 (1)	2 (2)	0 (0)
Professional Education			
Bachelor of Pharmacy (4 years)	245 (46)	47 (55)	239 (79)
Bachelor of Pharmacy (6 years)	257 (48)	-	-
Doctor of Pharmacy (PharmD)	-	21 (25)	32 (11)
Residency	-	-	3 (1)
Post-professional or post-baccalaureate PharmD	-	-	3 (1)
Master (M.Sc. or M.Pharm.)	23 (4)	12 (14)	20 (7)
Doctor of Philosophy (Ph.D.)	6 (1)	2 (2)	4 (1)

Table 3. *Cont.*

Characteristics	Japan (N = 534) *n* (%)	Thailand (N = 85) *n* (%)	Canada (N = 303) *n* (%)
Years of registration as a pharmacist			
<1 year	9 (2)	2 (2)	16 (5)
1–5 years	214 (40)	16 (19)	92 (30)
6–10 years	50 (9)	21 (25)	63 (21)
11–20 years	91 (17)	23 (27)	68 (22)
21–30 years	95 (18)	8 (9)	38 (13)
>31 years	74 (14)	15 (18)	25 (8)
Type of pharmacy			
Independent	68 (13)	67 (79)	83 (27)
Corporate/chain	322 (61)	12 (14)	172 (57)
Banner/franchise	1 (0)	6 (7)	44 (15)
Drugstore chain	135 (26)	-	-
Other	4 (1)	0 (0)	3 (1)

3.2. Provision of SRH Services

All categories of SRH services were, to some extent, provided in the three countries (Table 4). However, differences in involvement with the provision of these services were noted. In general, most participants from Thailand and Canada provided the services captured in the survey. Most of these participants reported dispensing combined hormonal contraceptives (Thailand = 99%, Canada = 98%) and emergency contraceptive pills (Thailand = 98%, Canada = 97%). Education on combined hormonal contraceptive methods, STBBI treatment, and maternal and perinatal health were also highly reported services (Thailand = 93–99%, Canada = 82–98%). Most Japanese participants provided patient education on barrier contraceptives for men (56%) and information on the safety of medications in pregnancy (74%) and breastfeeding (76%). A smaller number of Japanese participants provided and educated on emergency contraceptive pills (7% and 15%, respectively), educated patients on STBBI prevention (13%) and treatment (18%), and eighteen percent addressed the sexual health needs of lesbian, gay, bisexual, transgender, queer or questioning, intersex, asexual, and more (LGBTQ+) individuals.

Table 4. Sexual and reproductive health services provided by community pharmacists.

Service	Country		
	Japan (N = 534) *n* (%)	Thailand (N = 85) *n* (%)	Canada (N = 303) *n* (%)
1. Pregnancy Tests			
Patient education on pregnancy tests	192 (36)	83 (98)	211 (70)
2. Ovulation Tests			
Patient education on ovulation tests	222 (42)	70 (83)	152 (50)
3. Contraception			
Provide			
Combined hormonal contraceptives	250 (47)	84 (99)	298 (98)
Patient education on			
Combined hormonal contraceptives	207 (39)	84 (99)	295 (97)
Barrier contraception for men	299 (56)	67 (79)	210 (69)

Table 4. *Cont.*

Service	Country		
	Japan (N = 534) *n* (%)	**Thailand (N = 85)** *n* (%)	**Canada (N = 303)** *n* (%)
4. Emergency contraception			
Provision of EC pills (Levonorgestrel only pills, e.g., Plan B®)	37 (7)	82 (98)	294 (97)
Patient education on EC (Levonorgestrel only pills, e.g., Plan B®)	81 (15)	84 (99)	296 (98)
5. STBBI (chlamydia, gonorrhea, hepatitis B and C, genital herpes, syphilis, trichomoniasis, HIV, HPV)			
Patient education on STBBI treatment	96 (18)	82 (97)	247 (82)
Patient education on STBBI prevention	68 (13)	80 (94)	216 (71)
6. Maternal and perinatal health			
Patient education on nutrition and vitamin supplementation for prenatal and pregnancy care	253 (48)	79 (93)	278 (92)
Provision of information on safety of medications in pregnancy	395 (74)	85 (100)	297 (98)
Provision of information of recommended vaccines prior to and during pregnancy	139 (26)	39 (46)	259 (86)
Provision of information on safety of medications in breastfeeding	408 (76)	85 (100)	298 (98)
7. General Sexual Health			
Patient education on sexual dysfunction related to medications	159 (30)	51 (61)	255 (84)
Assist female patients identify/select options for sexual dysfunction	61 (11)	33 (39)	102 (34)
Assist male patients identify/select options for sexual dysfunction	67 (13)	53 (63)	207 (68)
Address sexual health concerns/needs of LGBTQ+ patients	95 (18)	40 (48)	132 (44)

EC, emergency contraception; STBBI, sexually transmitted and blood-borne infection; HIV, human immunodeficiency virus; HPV, human papillomavirus; LGBTQ+, lesbian, gay, bisexual, transgender, and queer (or questioning) and others.

3.3. Attitudes towards the Provision of SRH Professional Pharmacy Services

Overall, participants' attitudes in all three countries were positive toward pharmacists' roles in SRH (Figure 1). Most participants strongly agreed or agreed that offering advice on SRH is an essential part of community pharmacists' roles (Japan = 80%, Thailand = 95%, Canada = 93%) and that they had an ethical responsibility as pharmacists to provide SRH services (Japan = 67%, Thailand = 97%, Canada = 89%). Japanese participants were more likely to strongly disagree or disagree with statements regarding the need for SRH services in their local area (25%) and the use of SRH services by young people (56%). Sixty-four percent of Thai participants and 68% of Canadian participants believed pharmacists are adequately trained to provide SRH services, while over half of Japanese participants disagreed with this statement.

3.4. Perceived Factors Influencing the Provision of SRH Professional Pharmacy Services

In general, most participants from the three countries responded that all factors included in the survey influenced the provision of SRH services to some extent (Figure 2). In Japan, 93% of participants indicated pharmacists' knowledge "somewhat impacts the service" or "impacts the services to a great extent." Similarly, most Thai and Canadian participants highlighted the influence of pharmacists' knowledge (83% and 86% respectively). A higher percentage of all Canadian participants indicated pharmacy staffing (91%) influenced the provision of these services to a great extent, as compared to Japanese (74%) and Thai participants (80%). Compensation for the service "somewhat impact the service" or "impact the services to a great extent" for about half of participants in Japan and Thailand (56% and 46%, respectively), whereas for Canadian participants compensation had more impact on the provision of SRH services (77%).

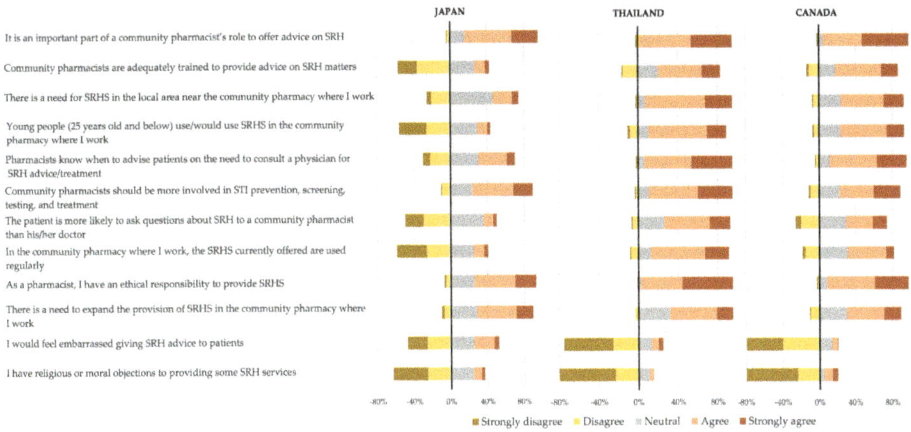

Figure 1. Comparison of attitudes towards the provision of sexual and reproductive health professional pharmacy services. (SRHS = Sexual and reproductive health services).

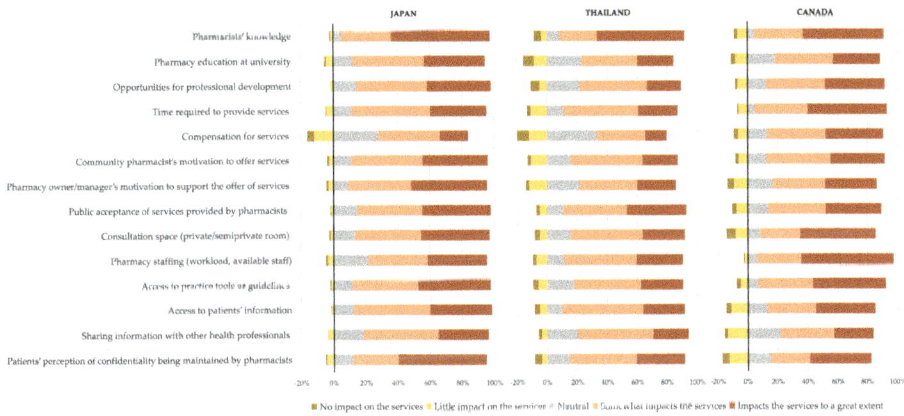

Figure 2. Comparison of perceived factors influencing the provision of sexual and reproductive health professional pharmacy services.

3.5. Preferences for Additional Training on SRH

Most respondents expressed interest in additional training in SRH services (Japan = 79%, Thailand = 91%, Canada = 84%). More than half of the participants in Japan (54%) and about three-quarters of the participants in Thailand and Canada (77% and 71%, respectively) were interested in expanding their roles in SRH.

Participants' preferences varied between countries. For Japanese participants interested in additional training, the top preferences were emergency contraception (77%) and hormonal contraceptives (63%), followed by pregnancy/postpartum/breastfeeding (59%). Additionally, the preferred areas for Thai participants were sexual dysfunction (68%), pregnancy/postpartum/breastfeeding (59%), and sexual health concerns of LGBTQ+ patients (55%). In Canada, approximately half of the participants or more preferred more training in the areas of STBBI treatment (64%), STBBI prevention (55%), and sexual health concerns of LGBTQ+ patients (50%) (Figure 3).

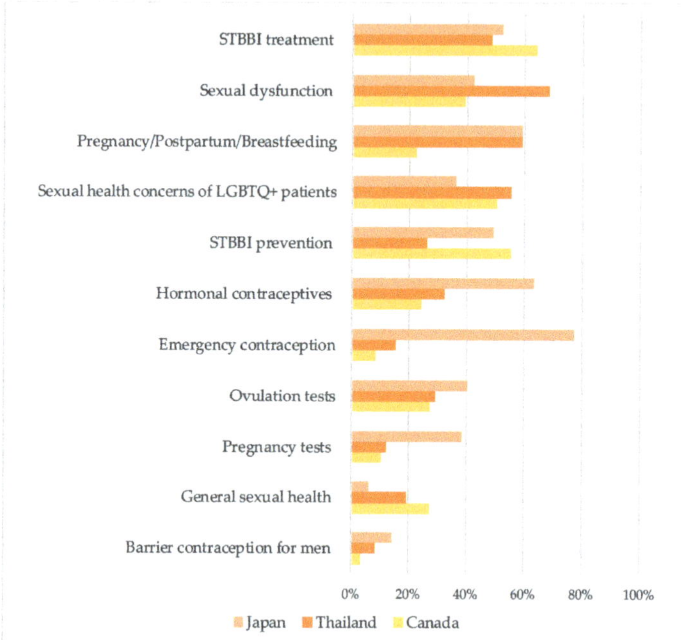

Figure 3. Comparison of preferences for additional training on sexual and reproductive health topics.

In terms of SRH competencies, more than 60% reported interest in additional training related to the use of appropriate and straightforward language when counselling patients (Japan = 70%, Thailand = 66%, Canada = 60%). This was the preferred choice for participants in Japan and Thailand, while for Canadian participants, their top selection was additional training on providing referrals (75%). Less than half of the participants reported interest in additional training related to confidentiality and privacy (Japan = 41%, Thailand = 31%, Canada = 29%). A higher proportion of Japanese participants considered approaching individuals nonjudgmentally a relevant topic for training (55%) (Figure 4).

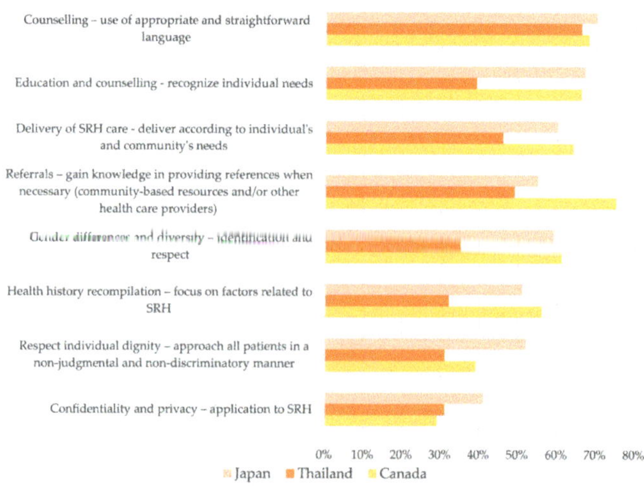

Figure 4. Comparison of training interests in sexual and reproductive health competencies.

4. Discussion

This multi-country study examined SRH services provided by pharmacists from regions with different regulations around pharmacy practice and perspectives regarding SRH. Results showed that pharmacists were involved in providing SRH services and had a positive attitude towards pharmacists' roles in SRH. Participants' perceptions of factors influencing the provision of SRH were similar in the three countries, as well as the willingness to expand roles and receive additional SRH training. The findings from this study can be used to inform education and training needs as well as potential barriers to the adoption of SRH services offered by community pharmacists.

Overall, a high percentage of Alberta pharmacists reported providing patient education across several SRH areas in addition to the provision of emergency contraception. This may be a reflection of changes in the scope of practice [57] and health policy and regulations in Alberta, Canada. In Thailand, pharmacy practice has evolved as well, and SRH services have been recognized as a pharmacy service [33]. Thai participants were highly involved with patient education in SRH, including emergency contraception and STBBI treatment and prevention. In Japan, the evolution of pharmacy practice has been more gradual compared to the other two countries [29,45]. In addition, sexual freedom, recognition of health risks, and access to SRH services are more recent public health concerns [31,58–60]. Overall, a lower percentage of Japanese participants provided SRH services included in this survey, including emergency contraception. Participants were more likely to report giving information related to the safety of medications in pregnancy and breastfeeding.

We found that community pharmacists from countries with different scopes of practice see themselves as SRH providers and consider offering advice on SRH topics an essential part of their roles. Still, they face similar challenges when providing SRH services. Regardless of differences in educational, economic, and healthcare system contexts, a set of competencies essential for patient care practice are similar in all regions [17,61]. Provision of SRH services, along with professional ethics and collaboration with patients and other health care providers, align with participants' views to meet patients' needs as SRH providers. All factors included in this survey were reported to influence the provision of SRH services to some extent. Knowledge of SRH, pharmacy staffing, and pharmacists' compensation were some of the main influencing factors for participants. Previous studies have identified barriers to implementing pharmacy services, including pharmacists' knowledge and the time required to provide the services [16,62].

One of the common findings was the willingness to receive more SRH training. However, the top preferences differed between countries, which can be influenced by the role participants associate with being an SRH provider. The focus of Japanese participants was emergency contraception, one of the main SRH discussion topics on the public agenda in Japan [30]. It is not surprising that Japanese pharmacists are interested in learning more about emergency contraception as their responsibilities have changed recently and will continue to change [52]. Alberta participants' primary preference was STBBI treatment. A syphilis outbreak was declared in 2019 [63]. Incidence rates of other sexually transmitted infections (chlamydia, gonorrhea) have continued to increase [64]. At the same time, the incidence of the human immunodeficiency virus (HIV) and hepatitis C virus (HCV) have not declined despite the availability of treatment and prevention tools [65]. In Thailand, sexual dysfunction was the most preferred topic for additional training. The high demand for medicines for sexual dysfunction [66,67], the challenges of their distribution (e.g., sildenafil is largely misused and is one of the most counterfeited drugs worldwide) [68], and the widespread use of herbal products with no scientific evidence for sexual health dysfunction may explain the preference of Thai participants.

To position pharmacists as SRH providers and increase access to SRH services, it is relevant that they see themselves as SRH providers. Recognizing that pharmacists' process to identify as SRH providers is dynamic, complex, and influenced by many factors will help to find the best tools and strategies to support their identity formation. Sharing international experiences on the influence of the changes in the profession can help to face challenges brought by this process. Exploring what different countries do to support their pharmacy workforce to prepare them to be SRH providers can inform the development of training programs and implementation strategies customized to the practice environment Expanding the offer of continuing education programs and creating pharmacist-specific guidelines and practice tools based on the context of each jurisdiction are some of the recommendations of this work.

Strengths and Limitations

The strengths of this study include the description of community pharmacists' perspectives regarding the provision of SRH services in Canada, Japan, and Thailand. This study is the first to characterize perceptions of SRH practice in several topics from pharmacists in countries with different scopes of practice. Despite these strengths, several limitations need to be considered. This study may not be generalized to other regions in the selected countries and nations. Due to our study design, the results are limited due to volunteer acquiescence, social desirability, and non-response bias. The sample size was not calculated a priori, and the number of participants varied between countries. No current detailed pharmacy workforce statistics are available to consider the representativeness of the population we aimed to survey in Japan and Thailand. However, the representativeness of this sample of the Canadian (Alberta) pharmacists' population has been described before [53]. The survey was developed and distributed during the COVID-19 pandemic, which impacted the distribution and recruitment processes, resulting in slightly different methods and timelines used in the three countries. In addition, the global health crisis may have affected pharmacists' workload and impacted our response rates.

5. Conclusions

Community pharmacists in countries with different scopes of practice and pharmacy regulations reported providing services in several SRH areas. While the extent to which pharmacists self-report the provision of SRH services varied in each country, pharmacists were interested in expanding SRH services and additional SRH training. Addressing factors that influence the provision of SRH services and supporting pharmacists is essential for expanding access. Sharing international experiences can guide challenges faced with the evolution of practice in SRH. Introducing support strategies based on local needs and international experiences, such as creating continuing education opportunities and practice tools, could help support pharmacists in providing care for individuals seeking SRH services.

Supplementary Materials: The following supporting information can be downloaded at: https://www.mdpi.com/article/10.3390/healthcare11111530/s1, File S1: SRH survey.

Author Contributions: Conceptualization, C.A.H., N.Y., T.J.S. and S.Y.; methodology, J.N., C.A.H., N.Y., T.J.S., S.Y., T.T., T.S., C.P. and P.A.; formal analysis, J.N. and C.A.H.; investigation, J.N.; data curation, J.N.; writing—original draft preparation, J.N. and C.A.H.; writing—review and editing, J.N., C.A.H., N.Y., T.J.S., S.Y., T.T., T.S., C.P. and P.A.; visualization, J.N. and C.A.H.; supervision, C.A.H.; project administration, C.A.H.; funding acquisition, C.A.H., N.Y., T.J.S. and S.Y. All authors have read and agreed to the published version of the manuscript.

Funding: This work was supported by the Faculty of Pharmacy and Pharmaceutical Sciences, University of Alberta (The Taiho Fund).

Institutional Review Board Statement: This study received approval from the Josai International University Research Ethics Review Committee (10M200001), the Chulalongkorn University Research Ethics Review Committee (114.1/63), and the University of Alberta Health Research Ethics Board (Pro00095881).

Informed Consent Statement: Informed consent was obtained from all subjects involved in the study.

Data Availability Statement: The data presented in this study are available on request from the corresponding author.

Acknowledgments: The authors wish to acknowledge the support of the EPICORE Centre and the Alberta SPOR Support Unit Consultation and Research Services in the online survey development and distribution, data management, and statistical services. JN acknowledges the National Agency for Research and Development (ANID)/Scholarship program for supporting her research (Master Becas Chile/2018—73190318).

Conflicts of Interest: The authors declare no conflict of interest.

References

1. World Health Organization. Sexual Health. Available online: https://www.who.int/topics/sexual_health/en/ (accessed on 10 April 2023).
2. Lindberg, L.D.; VandeVusse, A.; Mueller, J.; Kirstein, M. *Early Impacts of the COVID-19 Pandemic: Findings from the 2020 Guttmacher Survey of Reproductive Health Experiences*; Guttmacher Institute: New York, NY, USA, 2020. Available online: https://www.guttmacher.org/sites/default/files/report_pdf/early-impacts-covid-19-pandemic-findings-2020-guttmacher-survey-reproductive-health.pdf (accessed on 20 April 2023).
3. Dupuis, E.; Ali-Gami, J.; Wisofchi, S. *The Right to Sexual and Reproductive Health—Challenges and Possibilities during COVID 19: A Canadian Perspective*; International Youth Alliance for Family Planning Canada (IYAFP Canada): Ottawa, ON, Canada, 2021; pp. 1–19. Available online: https://www.ohchr.org/Documents/Issues/Health/sexual-reproductive-health-covid/CSOs/ngo.iyapfpdf.pdf (accessed on 20 April 2023).
4. Hussein, J. COVID-19: What implications for sexual and reproductive health and rights globally? *Sex. Reprod. Health Matters* **2020**, *28*, 1746065. [CrossRef] [PubMed]
5. Lindberg, L.; Bell, D.; Kantor, L. The sexual and reproductive health of adolescents and young adults during the COVID-19 pandemic. *Perspect. Sex. Reprod. Health* **2020**, *52*, 75–79. [CrossRef] [PubMed]
6. Tang, K.; Gaoshan, J.; Ahonsi, B.; Ali, M.; Bonet, M.; Broutet, N.; Kara, E.; Kim, C.; Thorson, A.; Thwin, S.S. Sexual and reproductive health (SRH): A key issue in the emergency response to the coronavirus disease (COVID-19) outbreak. *Reprod. Health* **2020**, *17*, 59. [CrossRef] [PubMed]
7. Church, K.; Gassner, J.; Elliott, M. Reproductive health under COVID-19—Challenges of responding in a global crisis. *Sex. Reprod. Health Matters* **2020**, *28*, 1773163. [CrossRef]
8. Wood, J.; Quinn-Nilas, C.; McKay, A.; Wentland, J. Perceived impact of COVID-19 on sexual health and access to sexual health services among university students in Canada. *Can. J. Hum. Sex.* **2022**, *31*, 79–90. [CrossRef]
9. VandeVusse, A.; Castillo, P.W.; Kirstein, M.; Mueller, J.; Kavanaugh, M. Disruptions and opportunities in sexual and reproductive health care: How COVID-19 impacted service provision in three US states. *Perspect. Sex. Reprod. Health* **2022**, *54*, 188–197. [CrossRef]
10. Morton, S.; Pencheon, D.; Squires, N. Sustainable Development Goals (SDGs), and their implementation: A national global framework for health, development and equity needs a systems approach at every level. *Br. Med. Bull.* **2017**, *124*, 81–90. [CrossRef]
11. Urick, B.Y.; Meggs, E.V. Towards a greater professional standing: Evolution of pharmacy practice and education, 1920–2020. *Pharmacy* **2019**, *7*, 98. [CrossRef]
12. Carmichael, J.M.; Hall, D.L. Evolution of ambulatory care pharmacy practice in the past 50 years. *Am. J. Health Syst. Pharm.* **2015**, *72*, 2087–2091. [CrossRef]
13. Clark, J.S.; Knoer, S.J.; Waier, K.A.; Montgomery, D.R.; Cesarz, J.; Chapman, N.R.M.; Kotis, D. Maximizing pharmacists' scope of practice. *Am. J. Health Syst. Pharm.* **2022**, *79*, 1397–1401. [CrossRef]
14. Weir, N.M.; Newham, R.; Dunlop, E.; Bennie, M. Factors influencing national implementation of innovations within community pharmacy: A systematic review applying the Consolidated Framework for Implementation Research. *Implement. Sci.* **2019**, *14*, 21. [CrossRef] [PubMed]
15. Gauly, J.; Ross, J.; Hall, I.; Soda, I.; Atherton, H. Pharmacy-based sexual health services: A systematic review of experiences and attitudes of pharmacy users and pharmacy staff. *Sex. Transm. Infect.* **2019**, *95*, 488–495. [CrossRef] [PubMed]
16. Navarrete, J.; Yuksel, N.; Schindel, T.J.; Hughes, C.A. Sexual and reproductive health services provided by community pharmacists: A scoping review. *BMJ Open* **2021**, *11*, e047034. [CrossRef]
17. International Pharmaceutical Federation. *FIP Report on Engagement with Our Membership 2021—Capturing the Voice of FIP Members Globally, to Advance Pharmacy Worldwide*; International Pharmaceutical Federation: The Hague, The Netherlands, 2022. Available online: https://www.fip.org/file/5157 (accessed on 4 April 2023).
18. Raza, M.A.; Aziz, S.; Noree, M.; Anjum, I.; Raza, S.M. A Portrait of the Pharmacy Profession Globally: Pharmacist Universal Professional Identity and Establishment of Global Pharmacy Council. *Innov. Pharm.* **2022**, *13*, 4. [CrossRef]
19. Bates, I.; Meilianti, S.; Bader, L.; Gandhi, R.; Leng, R.; Galbraith, K. Strengthening Primary Healthcare through accelerated advancement of the global pharmacy workforce: A cross-sectional survey of 88 countries. *BMJ Open* **2022**, *12*, e061860. [CrossRef] [PubMed]

20. International Pharmaceutical Federation (FIP). *Call to Action to Support Pharmacists and Pharmacy Workers on the Coronavirus COVID-19 Frontline*; International Pharmaceutical Federation: The Hague, The Netherlands, 2020; Available online: https://www.fip.org/files/content/publications/2020/FIP-call-to-action-to-support-pharmacists-and-pharmacy-workers-on-the-coronavirus-COVID-19-frontline.pdf (accessed on 30 March 2023).
21. Gilbert, M.; Chang, H.J.; Ablona, A.; Salway, T.; Ogilvie, G.S.; Wong, J.; Haag, D.; Pedersen, H.N.; Bannar-Martin, S.; Campeau, L.; et al. Accessing needed sexual health services during the COVID-19 pandemic in British Columbia, Canada: A survey of sexual health service clients. *Sex. Transm. Infect.* **2021**, *98*, 360–365. [CrossRef]
22. Kelly, D.V.; Kielly, J.; Hughes, C.; Gahagan, J.; Asghari, S.; Hancock, S.; Burt, K.; Smyczek, P.; Charlton, C.; Nguyen, H. Expanding access to HIV testing through Canadian community pharmacies: Findings from the APPROACH study. *BMC Public Health* **2020**, *20*, 639. [CrossRef]
23. Soon, J.A.; Whelan, A.M.; Yuksel, N.; Rafie, S. Enhancing access to contraception through pharmacist prescribing across Canada. *Can. Pharm. J.* **2021**, *154*, 356–362. [CrossRef]
24. Wong, K.R.; Hum, S.; McCarthy, L.; Dunn, S. Beyond Plan B: A qualitative study of Canadian pharmacists' emergency contraception counselling practices. *JOGC* **2017**, *39*, 1021–1027. [CrossRef]
25. Chanakit, T.; Low, B.Y.; Wongpoowarak, P.; Moolasarn, S.; Anderson, C. A survey of pharmacy education in Thailand. *Am. J. Pharm. Educ.* **2014**, *78*, 161. [CrossRef]
26. Supapaan, T.; Low, B.Y.; Wongpoowarak, P.; Moolasarn, S.; Anderson, C. A transition from the BPharm to the PharmD degree in five selected countries. *Pharm. Pract.* **2019**, *17*, 1611. [CrossRef] [PubMed]
27. Schindel, T.J.; Yuksel, N.; Hughes, C.A. Prescribing by Pharmacists. In *Encyclopedia of Evidence in Pharmaceutical Public Health and Health Services Research in Pharmacy*; University of Bath: Bath, UK, 2022; pp. 1–22.
28. Schindel, T.J.; Yuksel, N.; Breault, R.; Daniels, J.; Varnhagen, S.; Hughes, C.A. Pharmacists' learning needs in the era of expanding scopes of practice: Evolving practices and changing needs. *Res. Social. Adm. Pharm.* **2019**, *15*, 448–458. [CrossRef] [PubMed]
29. Nakagawa, S.; Kume, N. Pharmacy practice in Japan. *Can. J. Hosp. Pharm.* **2017**, *70*, 232–242. [CrossRef] [PubMed]
30. Kamijo, K.; Kataoka, Y.; Shigemi, D. Challenges of accessing emergency contraceptive pills in Japan. *BMJ Sex. Reprod. Health* **2021**, *47*, 232–233. [CrossRef] [PubMed]
31. Taniguchi, H.; Hisasue, S.I.; Sato, Y. Challenges in the practice of sexual medicine in the time of COVID-19 in Japan. *J. Sex. Med.* **2020**, *17*, 1237–1238. [CrossRef]
32. Nawanopparatsakul, S.; Keokitichai, S.; Wiyakarn, S.; Chantaraskul, C. Challenges of pharmacy education in Thailand. *Silpakorn Univ. Int. J.* **2010**, *9–10*, 19–39.
33. Jaisue, S. Pharmacy practice in Thailand. *J. Pharm. Pract. Res.* **2015**, *45*, 390–391. [CrossRef]
34. Regional Office for the Western Pacific. *The Kingdom of Thailand Health System Review*; WHO Regional Office for the Western Pacific: Manila, Philippines, 2015; p. 265. Available online: https://apps.who.int/iris/handle/10665/208216 (accessed on 25 March 2023).
35. Suwannaprom, P.; Suttajit, S.; Eakanunkul, S.; Supapaan, T.; Kessomboon, N.; Udomaksorn, K.; Sakulbumrungsil, R. Development of pharmacy competency framework for the changing demands of Thailand's pharmaceutical and health services. *Pharm. Pract.* **2020**, *18*, 2141. [CrossRef]
36. Panichkriangkrai, W.; Topothai, C.; Saengruang, N.; Thammatach-Aree, J.; Tangcharoensathien, V. Universal access to sexual and reproductive health services in Thailand: Achievements and challenges. *Sex. Reprod. Health Matters* **2020**, *28*, 1805842. [CrossRef]
37. Andajani, S.; Chanthasukh, S.; Fairbairn-Dunlop, P.; Smith, J.F. Community pharmacists' roles in providing contraceptive services: Views and experiences of adolescents in urban Khon Kaen, Northeast Thailand. *Int. J. Pharm. Pract.* **2023**, *31*, 276–281. [CrossRef]
38. Iguchi, K.; Ueyama, M.; Nishio, H.; Tamaki, H.; Osanai, A.; Ino, Y.; Nonomura, K.; Horibe, M.; Matsunaga, T.; Nakamura, M. Impact of the increase in the number of community pharmacists on their geographical distribution in Japan: A retrospective survey. *J. Pharm. Policy Pract.* **2022**, *15*, 96. [CrossRef] [PubMed]
39. National Association of Pharmacy Regulatory Authorities. National Statistics. Available online: https://www.napra.ca/resources/national-statistics/ (accessed on 30 March 2023).
40. The Pharmacy Council of Thailand. Number of Licensed Pharmacists to Practice Pharmacy Each Year. Available online: https://www.pharmacycouncil.org/index.php?option=content&menuid=33 (accessed on 30 March 2023).
41. Statista. Health, Pharma & Medtech. Available online: https://www.statista.com/markets/412/health-pharma-medtech/ (accessed on 30 March 2023).
42. Canadian Institute for Health Information. *Pharmacists in Canada, 2021—Data Tables*; CIHI: Ottawa, ON, Canada, 2022. Available online: https://www.cihi.ca/en/pharmacists (accessed on 30 March 2023).
43. Canadian Pharmacists Association. *CPhA Position Statement—Doctor of Pharmacy Degree as an Entry-Level to Practice*; Canadian Pharmacists Association: Toronto, ON, Canada, 2011. Available online: https://www.pharmacists.ca/cpha-ca/assets/File/cpha-on-the-issues/PharmD%20Entry%20Level.pdf (accessed on 20 April 2023).
44. Suttajit, S.; Suwannaprom, P.; Supapaan, T.; Eakanunkul, S.; Tangkiatkumjai, M.; Kongkaew, C.; Anderson, C.; Wongpoowarak, P. Are we on the right track? Answers from a national survey of Thai graduates' perceptions during the transition to the 6-year PharmD program. *Adv. Med. Educ. Pract.* **2018**, *9*, 713–722. [CrossRef] [PubMed]
45. Hasumoto, K.Y.; Thomas, R.K.; Yokoi, M.; Arai, K. Comparison of community pharmacy practice in Japan and US state of Illinois. *J. Pharm. Pract.* **2020**, *33*, 48–54. [CrossRef]

46. Chaiyakunapruk, N.; Jones, S.M.; Dhippayom, T.; Sumpradit, N. Pharmacy practice in Thailand. In *Pharmacy Practice in Developing Countries*; Elsevier: Amsterdam, The Netherlands, 2016; pp. 3–22.
47. Leelavanich, D.; Adjimatera, N.; Broese Van Groenou, L.; Anantachoti, P. Prescription and non-prescription drug classification systems across countries: Lessons learned for Thailand. *Risk Manag. Healthc. Policy* **2020**, *13*, 2753–2768. [CrossRef] [PubMed]
48. Utsumi, M.; Hirano, S.; Fujii, Y.; Yamamoto, H. Evaluation of the pharmacy practice program in the 6-year pharmaceutical education curriculum in Japan: Community pharmacy practice program. *J. Pharm. Health Care Sci.* **2015**, *1*, 27. [CrossRef] [PubMed]
49. Von Elm, E.; Altman, D.G.; Egger, M.; Pocock, S.J.; Gotzsche, P.C.; Vandenbroucke, J.P.; Initiative, S. The strengthening the reporting of observational studies in epidemiology (STROBE) statement: Guidelines for reporting observational studies. *J. Clin. Epidemiol.* **2008**, *61*, 344–349. [CrossRef] [PubMed]
50. Harris, P.A.; Taylor, R.; Thielke, R.; Payne, J.; Gonzalez, N.; Conde, J.G. Research electronic data capture (REDCap)—A metadata-driven methodology and workflow process for providing translational research informatics support. *J. Biomed. Inform.* **2009**, *42*, 377–381. [CrossRef]
51. Harris, P.A.; Taylor, R.; Minor, B.L.; Elliott, V.; Fernandez, M.; O'Neal, L.; McLeod, L.; Delacqua, G.; Delacqua, F.; Kirby, J.; et al. The REDCap consortium: Building an international community of software platform partners. *J. Biomed. Inform.* **2019**, *95*, 103208. [CrossRef]
52. Yamamura, S.; Terajima, T.; Navarrete, J.; Hughes, C.A.; Yuksel, N.; Schindel, T.J.; Sriboonruang, T.; Anantachoti, P.; Patikorn, C. Reproductive health services: Attitudes and practice of Japanese community pharmacists. *Healthcare* **2021**, *9*, 1336. [CrossRef]
53. Navarrete, J.; Hughes, C.A.; Yuksel, N.; Schindel, T.J.; Makowsky, M.J.; Yamamura, S. Community pharmacists' provision of sexual and reproductive health services: A cross-sectional study in Alberta, Canada. *J. Am. Pharm. Assoc.* **2022**, *62*, 1214–1223. [CrossRef]
54. Saleh, A.; Bista, K. Examining factors impacting online survey response rates in educational research: Perceptions of graduate students. *J. Multidiscip. Eval.* **2017**, *13*, 63–74. [CrossRef]
55. Blumenberg, C.; Menezes, A.M.B.; Gonçalves, H.; Assunção, M.C.F.; Wehrmeister, F.C.; Barros, F.C.; Barros, A.J.D. The role of questionnaire length and reminders frequency on response rates to a web-based epidemiologic study: A randomised trial. *Int. J. Soc. Res. Methodol.* **2019**, *22*, 625–635. [CrossRef]
56. Archer, T. Characteristics associated with increasing the response rates of web-based surveys. *Pract. Assess. Res. Eval.* **2007**, *12*, 12. [CrossRef]
57. Canadian Pharmacists Association. Pharmacists' Expanded Scope of Practice in Canada. Available online: https://www.pharmacists.ca/pharmacy-in-canada/scope-of-practice-canada/ (accessed on 2 April 2023).
58. Kodama, T.; Nakase, K.; Tsuda, T.; Yorifuji, T.; Doi, H. Factors affecting appropriate management of patients with sexually transmitted infections in Japan. *Acta Med. Okayama* **2010**, *64*, 171–179. [PubMed]
59. Ngatu, N.R.; Hirota, R.; Eitoku, M.; Muzembo, B.A.; Nishimori, M.; Kuramochi, M.; Shintani, S.; Inoue, S.; Takiuchi, R.; Maegawa, M.; et al. Perception of the risk of sexual transmission of HIV among Congolese and Japanese university students. *Environ. Health Prev. Med.* **2012**, *17*, 139–146. [CrossRef] [PubMed]
60. Ono-Kihara, M.; Kihara, M.; Yamazaki, H. Sexual practices and the risk for HIV/STDs infection of youth in Japan. *JMAJ* **2002**, *45*, 520–525.
61. Cappiello, J.; Levi, A.; Nothnagle, M. Core competencies in sexual and reproductive health for the interprofessional primary care team. *Contraception* **2016**, *93*, 438–445. [CrossRef]
62. Nordin, N.; Ahmad Hassali, M.A.; Sarriff, A. A global picture of extended pharmacy services, perceptions, and barriers toward its performance: A systematic review. *Asian J. Pharm. Clin. Res.* **2017**, *10*, 417–427. [CrossRef]
63. Alberta Health Services. Syphilis Outbreak, Information for Albertans. Available online: https://www.albertahealthservices.ca/info/Page17087.aspx (accessed on 15 March 2023).
64. Alberta Health Services. Alberta Sexually Transmitted Infections and HIV. 2020. Available online: https://open.alberta.ca/dataset/c6850032-20d3-4845-a465-568ed7e61b7c/resource/a50e1cd7-a968-480a-a4a4-332ddbf13597/download/health-alberta-sexually-transmitted-infections-and-hiv-2020.pdf (accessed on 20 April 2023).
65. Public Health Agency of Canada. *Report on Sexually Transmitted Infections in Canada, 2018*; Ministry of Health: Ottawa, ON, Canada, 2021. Available online: https://www.canada.ca/content/dam/hc-sc/documents/services/publications/diseases-conditions/report-sexually-transmitted-infections-canada/report-sexually-transmitted-infections-canada-2018.pdf (accessed on 30 March 2023).
66. Kongkanand, A.; Permpongkosol, S.; Tantiwongse, K. Thai men's health and sexual attitude. *Asian J. Androl.* **2011**, *13*, 534–536. [CrossRef]
67. Srithanaphakarangkul, K. Prevalence of sexual dysfunction and sexual attitudes among postmenopausal female patients in Phramongkutklao hospital. *J. Southeast Asian Med. Res.* **2019**, *3*, 82–87. [CrossRef]
68. Sansone, A.; Cuzin, B.; Jannini, E.A. Facing counterfeit medications in sexual medicine: A systematic scoping review on social strategies and technological solutions. *Sex. Med.* **2021**, *9*, 100437. [CrossRef] [PubMed]

healthcare MDPI

Article

Knowledge, Attitudes, and Practices among Pharmacy and Non-Pharmacy Interns in Saudi Arabia Regarding Antibiotic Use and Antibiotic Resistance: A Cross-Sectional Descriptive Study

Laila Albalawi [1], Abeer S. Alhawiti [1], Dania Alnasser [1], Jawaher Alhumaidi [1], Tahani Alrashidi [1], Awatif M. Alnawmasi [1], Mostafa A. S. Ali [2,3], Saleh Alqifari [2] and Hanan Alshareef [2,*]

[1] Faculty of Pharmacy, University of Tabuk, Tabuk 71491, Saudi Arabia
[2] Pharmacy Practice Department, Faculty of Pharmacy, University of Tabuk, Tabuk 71491, Saudi Arabia
[3] Department of Clinical Pharmacy, Faculty of Pharmacy, Assiut University, Assiut 71526, Egypt
[*] Correspondence: halsharef@ut.edu.sa

Abstract: This cross-sectional descriptive study aims to explore the knowledge, attitudes, and practices among pharmacy, dentistry, medicine, and nursing interns in Saudi Arabia regarding antibiotic use and antibiotic resistance. Interns received a soft copy of a structured and validated self-administered questionnaire using an online survey platform. A total of 266 interns responded to the questionnaire. On average, the participants achieved good scores in the knowledge and practice domains, followed by the attitude domain. The average knowledge percentage was 76.1% (SD 17.1) compared to 84.6% (SD 20.5) for practices and 61.5% (SD 23.2) for attitudes. The results suggest that pharmacy interns had insignificantly better overall scores compared to non-pharmacy interns for knowledge, attitudes, and practices. This study shows that the scores for knowledge, attitudes, and practices of pharmacy, dentistry, medicine, and nursing interns regarding antibiotic use and resistance were high overall. However, interns' belief in their responsibility in preventing antibiotic resistance is lacking.

Keywords: interns; antibiotics; antibiotic resistance; Saudi Arabia

check for updates

Citation: Albalawi, L.; Alhawiti, A.S.; Alnasser, D.; Alhumaidi, J.; Alrashidi, T.; Alnawmasi, A.M.; Ali, M.A.S.; Alqifari, S.; Alshareef, H. Knowledge, Attitudes, and Practices among Pharmacy and Non-Pharmacy Interns in Saudi Arabia Regarding Antibiotic Use and Antibiotic Resistance: A Cross-Sectional Descriptive Study. *Healthcare* **2023**, *11*, 1283. https://doi.org/10.3390/healthcare11091283

Academic Editors: Georges Adunlin and Tao-Hsin Tung

Received: 23 March 2023
Revised: 18 April 2023
Accepted: 28 April 2023
Published: 29 April 2023

1. Introduction

Antimicrobials are medications used to treat or prevent infectious diseases caused by microorganisms, including bacteria, viruses, fungi, and parasites [1]. Inappropriate use of antimicrobials results in the emergence of resistance, which is a serious condition that occurs when the microorganisms change over time and no longer respond to antimicrobials, making the infection harder to treat and increasing the risk of spread, the severity, and the mortality of the disease [2]. New resistance mechanisms are evolving and spreading worldwide, making common infectious diseases difficult to treat [2,3]. Antimicrobial resistance is increasing at an alarming rate worldwide, leading to higher hospital expenditures, lengths of stay, and increased healthcare costs for patients and their families [1,3].

At least 2.8 million individuals in the United States become infected with antimicrobial-resistant fungi or bacteria each year, with more than 35,000 people dying as a result [1,4]. According to the Centers for Disease Control and Prevention (CDC), antimicrobial resistance-related costs amount to more than USD 4.6 billion annually in the United States [4]. If the current trend of inappropriate and excessive antibiotic usage continues, it is anticipated that 10 million people will die worldwide by 2050 [5,6].

The scientific understanding of the issues linked to antibiotic use must be improved [7]. The majority of initiatives aiming to control the use of antimicrobials have focused on prescribers [4]. In Saudi Arabia, community pharmacists cannot dispense antibiotics without medical prescriptions; these regulatory policies were developed in response to the occurrence of widespread antimicrobial resistance and to improve antibiotic prescription procedures [7,8]. Antibiotic policies at the national and international levels and educational initiatives all form part of the guidelines, strategies, and instructional programs aimed to control antimicrobial use and reduce resistance [7,8]. The physician–patient relationship, clinical microbiology, health economics, and the most basic definitions of sickness and therapy are all important factors in antibiotic use [9].

Every healthcare member has particular responsibilities toward antibiotic stewardship [10]. Dentists write one in ten therapeutic antibiotic prescriptions in primary care, yet many of these prescriptions may be unneeded and exacerbate the critically important issue of bacterial resistance [11]. A study discovered that dentists' awareness of recommendations and indications for prescribing antibiotics was often rated as moderate. These investigations revealed that even when they are not required or suitable, antibiotic prescriptions are common [12,13]. The nurses' role is noted in several contexts, including in collaboration with other healthcare professionals, participation in prescribing choices, adherence to procedures, and patient and public education [14].

Future health workers should be educated about antimicrobial use and resistance during their undergraduate studies, and it is important to assess their knowledge and attitudes during their internship year [10]. They should have a well-developed awareness and adequate knowledge of antimicrobial resistance. Insufficient education on antimicrobial resistance may lead to serious medical problems for patients [10].

Many global studies have found areas of mistrust and knowledge gaps in prescribing antibiotics, and students recognize the need for additional learning and training in antimicrobial stewardship and prescribing [15]. Awareness and attitudes toward the correct usage of antibiotics between interns and other healthcare providers make a considerable difference in controlling antimicrobial resistance [16]. A previous study reported a high awareness of antimicrobial resistance among adult medical staff in Saudi Arabia [9]. According to previous studies, medical curricula focused on antibiotics' rational use significantly improved students' knowledge of antibiotics and discouraged inappropriate use of antibiotics in clinical practice [17]. In contrast, some studies concluded a low overall level of awareness of antibiotic use among residents in Saudi Arabia [18–20]. Many factors contribute to this level of awareness; among these factors is previous self-administration of antibiotics without a prescription. Additionally, lack of awareness is a major factor in the misuse of antibiotics worldwide [21].

Educating future practitioners on antibiotic use and antimicrobial stewardship is a global strategic goal. Promoting responsible antibiotic use is vital to limit the risk of antibiotic resistance [22,23]. However, it is critical to assess how effectively pharmacists, physicians, nurses, and dentists are educated and trained about antibiotics utilization in order to minimize the impacts of antimicrobial resistance on patient health. Currently, to the best of our knowledge, there is a lack of studies examining the perception of the above issues among pharmacy, medicine, nursing, and dental interns in Saudi Arabia. Therefore, this study aimed to evaluate the current pharmacy and non-pharmacy interns' knowledge, attitudes, and practices regarding antimicrobial resistance and antibiotic use in Saudi Arabia.

2. Materials and Methods

2.1. Study Design and Setting

A cross-sectional descriptive study was conducted between January and April 2022 in Saudi Arabia. A self-administered questionnaire was used to assess the knowledge, attitudes, and practices of antibiotic use and antimicrobial resistance among pharmacy and non-pharmacy interns. The data were collected using the online survey tool Google Forms.

2.2. Sample Size

The sample size was estimated using the Raosoft Sample Size Calculator (http://www.raosoft.com/samplesize.html) (accessed on 1 January 2022) based on a margin of error of 5%, a confidence level of 90%, a population size consisting of the number of pharmacy and non-pharmacy interns in the kingdom, and a response distribution of 50%. The calculated sample size was 266. The total sample was proportionally allocated based on the number of healthcare graduate students in Saudi universities according to the Ministry of Health statistic report of approximately 15,000 [24].

2.3. Study Population

The inclusion criteria included pharmacy and non-pharmacy interns (medicine, dentistry, and nursing) who graduated from governmental or private Saudi universities.

The exclusion criteria included interns who had completed their internship year.

2.4. Data Collection Tool

Pharmacy and non-pharmacy interns received a soft copy of the survey questionnaire using the online survey platform Google Forms. After reviewing the literature [25–27] reporting on awareness and attitudes toward antibiotic use, we adopted the currently presented validated questionnaire because it has three different domains addressing the knowledge, attitudes, and practices of antibiotics. Each domain comprised professional questions inquiring about antibiotic consumption, perceptions, and general practice. The questionnaire was then reviewed by a faculty member expert in the field from the University of Tabuk to assess each domain's component, content, clarity, relevance, and comprehensibility.

The questionnaire consisted of two sections. The first explored participants' demographics, including gender, profession, college, and region. The second evaluated the interns' knowledge, attitudes, and practices concerning antibiotic prescriptions and antimicrobial resistance. The second part had 3 domains; the knowledge domain was assessed using 15 items, the attitude domain was assessed using 8 items, and the third domain assessed practices on 5 items. All questions were close-ended, and participants' responses were obtained for the knowledge and attitude domains on a 3-point response scale (agree, disagree, and not sure). The response to the practice domain was assessed through yes or no responses. The correct response to each question carried one mark. The overall score was graded as poor ($\leq$50%), adequate (from 51 to <75%), or good $\geq$75% depending on the percentage of correct responses.

2.5. Ethical Considerations

The local Research Ethics Committee at the University of Tabuk officially approved this study (approval number, UT-186-41-2022). Informed consent was obtained from all participants.

2.6. Statistical Analysis

The internal consistency and reliability of the questionnaire were examined by calculating Cronbach's alpha coefficient. The antibiotics questionnaire had a good internal consistency (Cronbach's α = 0.81). The standard descriptive analysis was summarized to describe the demographic characteristics of the participants. A bivariate analysis using chi-square or Fisher exact test, when appropriate, was used to generate p values of the percentages of the correct responses for each item of the questionnaire between pharmacy and non-pharmacy interns. A p value of less than 0.05 was considered statistically significant. The sum scores of the correct responses per participant on each of the knowledge, attitude, and practice domains of antibiotic use were calculated. Then, the mean proportions and standard deviations of the three scores were calculated and tested for pharmacy and non-pharmacy interns using the Wilcoxon–Mann–Whitney test. The Spearman's rank correlation was used to measure the direction of association between interns' knowledge and their practices of antibiotic use.

All analyses were carried out using STATA SE V.11 (Stata Corp, College Station, TX, USA).

3. Results

3.1. Interns' Demographic Characteristics and the Overall Average Score

A total of 266 respondents agreed to participate in this study, of whom 140 (52.6%) were male, and 244 (91.7%) attended governmental universities. The majority of participants were pharmacy interns (124, 46.6%), while 142 participants (53.4%) were interns at non-pharmacy schools, including schools in the medicine (87; 32.7%), dentistry (40; 15%), and nursing (15; 5.7%) domains. Many interns were from the middle region (76 interns; 28.5%) and the south region (62 interns; 23.3%). The characteristics of the study participants are illustrated in Table 1.

Table 1. Respondents' demographic characteristics (n = 266).

Variables		Frequency	Percentage (%)
Gender	Male	140	52.6
	Female	126	47.4
Profession	Pharmacy	124	46.6
	Medicine	87	32.7
	Dentistry	40	15
	Nursing	15	5.7
Region	North	51	19.1
	East	35	13.1
	West	43	16.1
	Middle	76	28.5
	South	62	23.3
Type of University	Governmental	244	91.7
	Private	22	8.3

The average percentages of correct scores for pharmacy interns compared with non-pharmacy interns on the knowledge, attitude, and practice domains of the antibiotic use questionnaire are illustrated in (Table 2). The distribution of participants' average scores in each domain of the questionnaire is shown in (Table 2).

Table 2. Pharmacy and non-pharmacy interns' average correct scores on the knowledge, attitude, and practice domains of antibiotic use.

Domain	Total n = 266	Pharmacy n = 124	Non-Pharmacy n = 142	p Value *
		Mean score % (SD)		
Knowledge	76.1 (17.1)	78.3 (14.8)	74.2 (18.6)	0.13
Attitude	61.5 (23.2)	63.7 (23.1)	59.5 (23.3)	0.11
Practice	84.6 (20.5)	84.8 (21.4)	84.6 (19.8)	0.55

* Significant p value < 0.05.

On average, interns demonstrated good scores (≥75% correct response) on the knowledge and practice domains of the questionnaire and adequate scores (51–75% correct response) on attitude toward antibiotic use. The analysis showed that pharmacy interns demonstrated higher but insignificant differences in the percentage of correct scores on the knowledge, attitude, and practice domains of antibiotic use of the questionnaire. The percentage of correct responses for each item of the questionnaire is illustrated in Tables 3–5.

Table 3. Frequency and percentage of correct responses for knowledge items.

Knowledge Items (Correct Response)	Pharmacy n = 124 (%)	Non-Pharmacy n = 142 (%)	Total n = 266 (%)	p Value *
1. Antibiotics are used to treat viral infections (D)	105 (84.7)	130 (91.6)	235 (88.4)	0.08
2. Antibiotics are useful against all types of common cold (D)	108 (87.1)	126 (88.7)	234 (87.7)	0.68
3. Clinical samples should be sent to culture and sensitivity before starting antibiotics (A)	86 (69.4)	94 (66.2)	180 (67.7)	0.58
4. The efficacy is better if the antibiotics are newer and more costly (D)	92 (74.2)	93 (65.5)	185 (69.5)	0.12
5. Antibiotics cause negative effects on the body's own bacterial flora (A)	97 (78.2)	114 (80.3)	211 (79.3)	0.68
6. Incomplete antibiotic intake contributes to antibiotic resistance (A)	115 (92.7)	124 (87.3)	239 (89.9)	0.15
7. Inaccurate antibiotic selection contributes to antibiotic resistance (A)	112 (91.1)	115 (80.9)	277 (85.7)	0.02 *
8. Inadequate dosage of antibiotics contributes to antibiotic resistance (A)	107 (86.3)	114 (80.3)	221 (83.1)	0.19
9. Overprescription of antibiotics contributes to antibiotic resistance (A)	114 (91.9)	112 (85.9)	236 (88.7)	0.12
10. Overconsumption of antibiotics contributes to antibiotic resistance (A)	106 (85.5)	108 (76.1)	214 (80.5)	0.05
11. Nosocomial infection spread contributes to antibiotic resistance (A)	73 (58.9)	64 (44.1)	137 (51.5)	0.03 *
12. Self-medication of antibiotics contributes to antibiotic resistance (A)	107 (86.3)	113 (79.6)	220 (82.7)	0.15
13. Frequent use of same antibiotic will reduce the efficacy of the treatment (A)	78 (62.9)	98 (69.0)	176 (66.2)	0.29
14. Unnecessary use of antibiotics can lead to antibiotic resistance (A)	114 (91.9)	125 (88.0)	239 (89.9)	0.29
15. Antibiotic resistance can spread from animals to humans (A)	43 (34.9)	40 (28.2)	83 (31.2)	0.25

Note: (A) Agree, (D) Disagree. * Significant p value < 0.05.

Table 4. Frequency and percentages of positive attitudes toward antimicrobial prescribing and resistance.

Attitude Items (Correct Response)	Pharmacy n = 124 (%)	Non-Pharmacy n =142 (%)	Total n = 266 (%)	p Value *
16. Antibiotics are safe drugs and, hence, can be commonly used (D)	94 (75.8)	92 (64.8)	186 (69.9)	0.071
17. Irrational antibiotic practice locally will not matter for global resistance (D)	88 (71.0)	104 (73.2)	192 (72.1)	0.68
18. Skipping one or two doses does not contribute to antibiotic resistance (D)	83 (66.9)	87 (61.2)	170 (63.9)	0.34

Table 4. *Cont.*

Attitude Items (Correct Response)	Pharmacy $n = 124$ (%)	Non-Pharmacy $n = 142$ (%)	Total $n = 266$ (%)	p Value *
19. Antibiotic resistance can be reduced using higher antibiotics in spite of lower antibiotics being sensitive (D)	71 (57.3)	64 (45.1)	135 (50.8)	0.047 *
20. Medical experts will solve the problem of antibiotic resistance before it becomes too serious (D)	21 (16.9)	19 (13.4)	40 (15.1)	0.42
21. There is not much people, like me, can do to stop antibiotic resistance (D)	56 (45.2)	72 (50.7)	128 (48.1)	0.37
22. Adhering to antibiotic policy of the hospital will reduce the development of antibiotic resistance (A)	108 (87.1)	123 (86.6)	231 (86.8)	0.91
23. Antibiotic resistance is one of the biggest problems the world faces (A)	111 (89.5)	115 (80.9)	226 (85.0)	0.052

Note: (A) Agree, (D) Disagree. * Significant p value < 0.05.

Table 5. Participant's self-reported practices regarding antibiotic use.

Practice Items (Correct Response)	Pharmacy $n = 124$ (%)	Non-Pharmacy $n = 142$ (%)	Total $n = 266$ (%)	p Value *
24. Do you consult a doctor before starting an antibiotic? (Yes)	117 (94.4)	124 (87.3)	241 (90.6)	0.05
25. Do you prescribe the same antibiotic for relatives/friends for similar illnesses without consulting the doctor? (No)	105 (84.7)	120 (84.5)	225 (84.6)	0.97
26. Do you pressurize the doctor to prescribe antibiotics? (No)	98 (79.0)	122 (85.9)	220 (85.9)	0.14
27. Do you complete the full course of antibiotics treatment? (Yes)	109 (87.9)	118 (83.1)	227 (85.3)	0.27
28. Do you save the remaining antibiotics for the next time you get sick? (No)	97 (78.2)	116 (81.7)	213 (80.1)	0.48

* Significant p value < 0.05.

3.2. Knowledge of Antibiotic Use and Antibiotic Resistance

The pattern of average scores on each item of the knowledge domain showed that pharmacy interns achieved a higher percentage of correct responses than non-pharmacy medical interns. The scores of pharmacy interns were significantly higher for some questions inquiring about the association between the development of antibiotic resistance and appropriate antibiotic selection ($p = 0.02$) and the spread of nosocomial infection ($p = 0.03$). Pharmacy interns were more likely to be aware of the contribution of overconsumption of antibiotics to antibiotic resistance ($p = 0.05$). Two-thirds of interns (183; 68.8%) reported poor knowledge and confusion about whether antibiotic resistance can spread from animals to humans in question 15 without significant differences between professions.

3.3. Attitude of Interns toward Antibiotic Use and Antibiotic Resistance

A similar pattern of average correct responses was observed for questions regarding the attitude of interns toward antimicrobial prescription. The majority of responses reported a highly positive attitude among all professions. A negative attitude was observed toward the sole role of medical experts in solving antibiotic resistance issues. The average attitude score for all interns was adequate at 61.5%.

3.4. Practices of Interns Regarding Antibiotic Use and Antibiotic Resistance

The average practice score showed a good response (85.3%). Self-reported practices were appropriate, and there was no significant difference between pharmacy and non-pharmacy interns (Table 5).

The weakly positive and significant correlation between the percentage of correct scores on the practices of participants regarding antibiotic use and their score on knowledge of the use of antibiotics is illustrated in Figure 1 (Spearman's rho = 0.32; $p = 0.001$).

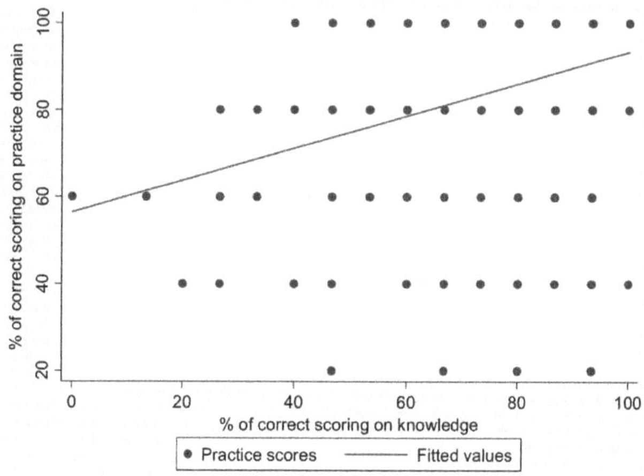

Figure 1. Correlation between percentage of correct scores on practice domain based on scores on knowledge.

4. Discussion

Globally, educating future healthcare professionals about antimicrobial use and resistance is a strategic objective [23]. With the increased occurrence of antibiotic prescriptions during the COVID-19 era, encouraging the responsible use of antibiotics is crucial to reduce the risk of antimicrobial resistance, and healthcare professionals are involved in the prescription, dispensing, administration, and use of antibiotics [22,28]. To reduce the negative effects of antimicrobial resistance on patients' health, it is crucial to evaluate how well future pharmacists, physicians, nurses, and dentists are educated and trained on the proper use of antibiotics.

This cross-sectional study assessed the awareness, attitudes, and practices of pharmacy and non-pharmacy interns, including medicine, dentistry, and nursing interns, regarding antibiotic use and antibiotic resistance in Saudi Arabia. To the best of our knowledge, this is the first study in Saudi Arabia to assess interns' knowledge of antibiotic use and antibiotic resistance. We chose interns as the participants in our study as they are future healthcare practitioners who will prescribe, dispense, monitor, and administer antibiotics. Assessing their awareness levels will help improve practices and minimize antibiotic misuse and resistance.

Our results reveal overall good levels of knowledge (76.1%) and practice (84.6%) and adequately positive attitudes (61.5%) among interns in Saudi Arabia, which reflect a satisfactory level of material in undergraduate curricula about antibiotic use and mechanism and causes of antimicrobial resistance.

In the current study, pharmacy interns had higher but insignificant scores in the knowledge domain than non-pharmacy interns. The scores of pharmacy interns were significantly higher for some questions inquiring about appropriate antibiotic selection, the spread of nosocomial infection, and the development of antibiotic resistance. A cross-sectional study was conducted to assess the infectious disease contents in pharmacy curricula at Saudi universities, including material on antibiotic use and antimicrobial stewardship [29]. They found that crucial infectious disease topics were covered in the curriculum by 78% of Saudi pharmacy colleges. These topics should prepare and enable graduates from these programs to enact better practices and provide better patient-centered care. This may also imply that pharmacists are distinctively qualified medical professionals who can play essential roles in the fight against antimicrobial misuse and resistance if they are involved in regulatory policies and educational interventions.

In this study, although all interns scored and expressed a good level of knowledge about antibiotic use, poor to adequate responses were reported for three questions regarding sending clinical samples before starting antibiotics, the efficacy of new antibiotics, and the spread of nosocomial infection. Unfortunately, our study showed that two-thirds of interns had poor knowledge and confusion about whether antibiotic resistance can spread from animals to humans. Similar results were reported by a previous study conducted in India, including medical interns [25]. This poor knowledge about the spread of antibiotic resistance from animals to humans demonstrates the need to promote awareness of this phenomenon in undergraduate curricula. At this stage, knowledge of antibiotics should be promoted through training, clinical rotations, or awareness workshops and activities. However, the knowledge of antibiotic use among medical students from different countries reported in the literature demonstrated variable results. Studies conducted in Colombia [26] and the United Arab of Emirates (UAE) [30] reported lower scores of knowledge among medical students, while a study conducted in Jordan reported a higher score (>75%) for students' knowledge of antibiotic use and resistance [31]. This variation in the knowledge scores observed between different studies may be attributed to differences in the presence of materials about antimicrobials in curricula among universities and the recruited students' performance and sociodemographic characteristics. However, the validated questionnaires used in these studies assessed the knowledge on antibiotic use and resistance; the minimal differences in the content may be a reason for the differences in the knowledge between the studies [26,30,31].

In the current study, despite the good knowledge of the participating interns, they had adequate scores for attitudes toward antibiotic use (61.5%). Moreover, some responses showed negative attitudes; half of the respondents believed that antibiotic resistance can be reduced by using broader-spectrum antibiotics and that they do not have a pivotal role in controlling the resistance, and 85% of the participants agreed that medical experts will solve the problem of antibiotic resistance before it becomes too serious. Adequate responses (51–75%) were scored for items related to the use of antibiotics and irrational practice. Similar attitudes were reported from studies conducted in India on medical students and interns [25] and medical students in Columbia [26]. However, a study conducted in Jordan on medical, pharmacy, and nursing students reported positive attitudes and that 62.8% of the participants believed that they have a role in controlling antibiotic resistance [31], and another study showed highly positive attitudes with a score of 80% among medical students in the United Arab Emirates (UAE) [30]. Pharmacy and medical schools in Saudi Arabia should offer more support to their undergraduate students by delivering more appropriate, well-designed curricula that address the proper use of antibiotics and the global risk of antimicrobial resistance. This will help promote the confidence of professional healthcare providers in dealing with antibiotics.

Regarding self-reported practices in this study, all interns expressed good levels with an average score of more than 80%, and there was no significant difference between pharmacy and non-pharmacy interns. However, our study showed that there was a positive correlation between the knowledge of interns and their practices of antibiotic use. This reflects the pharmacy and medical interns' readiness to implement their awareness and beliefs in practice. On the other hand, a cross-sectional study conducted in Spain to identify factors that affect antibiotic prescribing practices among medical interns demonstrated the judgment of the attending physician was the main factor affecting medical interns' antibiotic prescribing practices in this study [32].

Our study addressed the awareness and attitudes of pharmacy and non-pharmacy interns who shared many demographic characteristics, such as age, Saudi nationality, and socioeconomic status. The majority (92%) were enrolled in governmental universities and had limited experience in dealing with antibiotics, with the exception of their advanced training year. The demographic variable that was hypothesized to influence their awareness and attitudes toward antibiotic use was the undergraduate educational program (profession). Therefore, the study focused on this variable in the analysis. Moreover, the findings of the univariate analysis revealed no significant differences in the average scores of each domain, so a multivariate analysis was not necessary.

This study has the strength of being the first study to assess interns' knowledge, attitudes, and practices regarding antibiotic use and resistance in Saudi Arabia. These interns are in their initial steps of professional practice. However, the current study has some limitations that should be acknowledged, mainly related to the study design. A cross-sectional survey design limited our ability to identify factors affecting the awareness and beliefs of interns. The small sample size of participants from different universities is another limitation. Third, the self-report scale used for data collection may lead to recall bias. The participants might overestimate some socially desirable attitudes or practices regarding antibiotic use.

5. Conclusions

The current study demonstrates that the knowledge, attitudes, and practices regarding antibiotic use and resistance among pharmacy and non-pharmacy interns in Saudi Arabia are adequate overall. In addition, knowledge was positively correlated with interns experience in practices related to antibiotic use. However, interns' attitude toward their role and responsibility regarding the spread of antibiotic resistance is lacking. Further studies are needed to identify areas and effective means of development for pharmacy and non-pharmacy interns in Saudi Arabia.

Author Contributions: Conceptualization, L.A., A.S.A. and T.A.; methodology, A.M.A. and T.A.; validation, M.A.S.A., D.A. and J.A.; formal analysis, M.A.S.A.; data curation, D.A.; writing—original draft preparation, L.A., A.S.A., T.A., A.M.A., D.A. and J.A.; writing—review and editing, M.A.S.A., S.A. and H.A.; visualization, M.A.S.A., S.A. and H.A.; supervision, H.A.; project administration, S.A. and H.A.; funding acquisition, H.A. All authors have read and agreed to the published version of the manuscript.

Funding: This research was funded by the Deanship of Scientific Research, University of Tabuk, Tabuk, Saudi Arabia, grant number (0083-1443-S).

Institutional Review Board Statement: The study was conducted in accordance with the Declaration of Helsinki, and the local Research Ethics Committee at the University of Tabuk officially approved this study (approval number, UT-186-41-2022).

Informed Consent Statement: Informed consent was obtained from all subjects involved in the study.

Data Availability Statement: Data are available upon request from the corresponding author.

Conflicts of Interest: The authors declare no conflict of interest. The funders had no role in the design of the study; in the collection, analyses, or interpretation of data; in the writing of the manuscript; or in the decision to publish the results.

References

1. World Health Organization. Antimicrobial Resistance. Available online: https://www.who.int/news-room/fact-sheets/detail/antimicrobial-resistance (accessed on 18 April 2022).
2. Ventola, C.L. The antibiotic resistance crisis: Part 1: Causes and threats. *Pharm. Ther.* **2015**, *40*, 277–283.
3. Prestinaci, F.; Pezzotti, P.; Pantosti, A. Antimicrobial resistance: A global multifaceted phenomenon. *Pathog. Glob. Health* **2015**, *109*, 309–318. [CrossRef] [PubMed]
4. Centers for Disease Control and Prevention. Antibiotic Resistance Threats in the United States. 2019. Available online: https://www.cdc.gov/drugresistance/biggest-threats.html (accessed on 10 February 2022).

5. Pulingam, T.; Parumasivam, T.; Gazzali, A.M.; Sulaiman, A.M.; Chee, J.Y.; Lakshmanan, M.; Chin, C.F.; Sudesh, K. Antimicrobial resistance: Prevalence, economic burden, mechanisms of resistance and strategies to overcome. *Eur. J. Pharm. Sci.* **2022**, *170*, 106103. [CrossRef] [PubMed]
6. Shinu, P.; Mouslem, A.K.A.; Nair, A.B.; Venugopala, K.N.; Attimarad, M.; Singh, V.A.; Nagaraja, S.; Alotaibi, G.; Deb, P.K. Progress Report: Antimicrobial Drug Discovery in the Resistance Era. *Pharmaceuticals* **2022**, *15*, 413. [CrossRef]
7. Alhomoud, F.; Almahasnah, R.; Alhomoud, F.K. "You could lose when you misuse"—Factors affecting over-the-counter sale of antibiotics in community pharmacies in Saudi Arabia: A qualitative study. *BMC Health. Serv. Res.* **2018**, *18*, 915. [CrossRef] [PubMed]
8. MOH News. MOH Warns Against Selling Antibiotics without Prescription. April 2018. Available online: https://www.moh.gov.sa/en/Ministry/MediaCenter/News/Pages/news-2018-04-17-004.aspx (accessed on 1 January 2022).
9. Al-Shibani, N.; Hamed, A.; Labban, N.; Al-Kattan, R.; Al-Otaibi, H.; Alfadda, S. Knowledge, attitude and practice of antibiotic use and misuse among adults in Riyadh, Saudi Arabia. *Saudi Med. J.* **2017**, *38*, 1038–1044. [CrossRef]
10. Akbar, Z.; Alquwez, N.; Alsolais, A.; Thazha, S.K.; Ahmad, M.D.; Cruz, J.P. Knowledge about antibiotics and antibiotic resistance among health-related students in a Saudi University. *J. Infect. Dev. Ctries.* **2021**, *15*, 925–933. [CrossRef]
11. Johnson, T.M.; Hawkes, J. Awareness of antibiotic prescribing and resistance in primary dental care. *Prim. Dent. J.* **2014**, *3*, 44–47. [CrossRef]
12. Halboub, E.; Alzaili, A.; Quadri, M.F.; Al-Haroni, M.; Al-Obaida, M.I.; Al-Hebshi, N.N. Antibiotic Prescription Knowledge of Dentists in Kingdom of Saudi Arabia: An Online, Country-wide Survey. *J. Contemp. Dent. Pract.* **2016**, *17*, 198–204. [CrossRef]
13. Shati, A.A. Dentists' knowledge and practices about infective endocarditis antibiotics prophylaxis among children in aseer region, Southwestern Saudi Arabia. *Niger. J. Clin. Pract.* **2022**, *25*, 123–129. [CrossRef]
14. Davey, K.; Aveyard, H. Nurses' perceptions of their role in antimicrobial stewardship within the hospital environment. An integrative literature review. *J. Clin. Nurs.* **2022**, *31*, 3011–3020. [CrossRef]
15. Efthymiou, P.; Gkentzi, D.; Dimitriou, G. Knowledge, Attitudes and Perceptions of Medical Students on Antimicrobial Stewardship. *Antibiotics* **2020**, *9*, 821. [CrossRef]
16. Mersha, A. Attitude and perception of medical interns about antimicrobial resistance: A multi center cross-sectional study in Ethiopia. *Antimicrob. Resist. Infect. Control* **2018**, *7*, 149. [CrossRef]
17. Zaidi, S.F.; Alotaibi, R.; Nagro, A.; Alsalmi, M.; Almansouri, H.; Khan, M.A.; Khan, A.; Memon, I. Knowledge and Attitude Towards Antibiotic Usage: A Questionnaire-Based Survey Among Pre-Professional Students at King Saud bin Abdulaziz University for Health Sciences on Jeddah Campus, Saudi Arabia. *Pharmacy* **2020**, *8*, 5. [CrossRef]
18. Memon, I.; Alrashid, A.A.; Alshammari, H.S.; Rehman, D.-e.-S.; Feroz, Z.; Nagro, A.; Alotaibi, R.; Alsalmi, M.; Khan, M.A.; Alkushi, A.; et al. Assessing the Effects of Basic Medical Science Courses on the Knowledge and Attitude towards Antibiotic Usage among Pre-Professional Students in Saudi Arabia. *Pharmacy* **2021**, *9*, 108. [CrossRef]
19. Benmerzouga, I.; Al-Zammay, S.A.; Al-Shammari, M.M.; Alsaif, S.A.; Alhaidan, T.M.; Aljofan, M. Practices of patients consuming antibiotics and knowledge about antibiotic resistance in Hail region—Saudi Arabia. *Future Sci. OA* **2019**, *5*, FSO420. [CrossRef]
20. El Zowalaty, M.E.; Belkina, T.; Bahashwan, S.A.; El Zowalaty, A.E.; Tebbens, J.D.; Abdel-Salam, H.A.; Khalil, A.I.; Daghriry, S.I.; Gahtani, M.A.; Madkhaly, F.M.; et al. Knowledge, awareness, and attitudes toward antibiotic use and antimicrobial resistance among Saudi population. *Int. J. Clin. Pharm.* **2016**, *38*, 1261–1268. [CrossRef]
21. Alnasser, A.H.A.; Al-Tawfiq, J.A.; Ahmed, H.A.A.; Alqithami, S.M.H.; Alhaddad, Z.M.A.; Rabiah, A.S.M.; Albrahim, M.A.A.; Al Kalif, M.S.H.; Barry, M.; Temsah, M.H.; et al. Public Knowledge, Attitude and Practice towards Antibiotics Use and Antimicrobial Resistance in Saudi Arabia: A Web-Based Cross-Sectional Survey. *J. Public Health Res.* **2021**, *10*, 2276. [CrossRef]
22. Cantón, R.; Akova, M.; Langfeld, K.; Torumkuney, D. Relevance of the Consensus Principles for Appropriate Antibiotic Prescribing in 2022. *J. Antimicrob. Chemother.* **2022**, *77*, i2–i9. [CrossRef]
23. World Health Organization. *Health Workers' Education and Training on Antimicrobial Resistance: Curricula Guide*; World Health Organization: Geneva, Switzerland, 2019.
24. Ministry of Health: Statistical Year Book. 2018. Available online: https://www.moh.gov.sa/en/Ministry/Statistics/book/Documents/book-Statistics.pdf (accessed on 14 December 2021).
25. Ningappa, A.; Dhanalakshmi, T.; Shyamanth, M. Knowledge, attitude, and practices toward antibiotic usage and antibiotic resistance among medical students and interns: A cross-sectional study. *J. Med. Sci. Health* **2020**, *6*, 12–17. [CrossRef]
26. Higuita-Gutiérrez, L.F.; Roncancio Villamil, G.E.; Jiménez Quiceno, J.N. Knowledge, attitude, and practice regarding antibiotic use and resistance among medical students in Colombia: A cross-sectional descriptive study. *BMC Public Health* **2020**, *20*, 1861. [CrossRef]
27. Ashiru-Oredope, D.; Hopkins, S.; Vasandani, S.; Umoh, E.; Oloyede, O.; Nilsson, A.; Kinsman, J.; Elsert, L.; Monnet, D.L.; #ECDC Antibiotic Survey Project Advisory Group. Healthcare workers' knowledge, attitudes and behaviours with respect to antibiotics, antibiotic use and antibiotic resistance across 30 EU/EEA countries in 2019. *Eurosurveillance* **2021**, *26*, 1900633. [CrossRef]
28. Perrella, A.; Fortinguerra, F.; Pierantozzi, A.; Capoluongo, N.; Carannante, N.; Lo Vecchio, A.; Bernardi, F.F.; Trotta, F.; Cangini, A. Hospital Antibiotic Use during COVID-19 Pandemic in Italy. *Antibiotics* **2023**, *12*, 168. [CrossRef]
29. Alqahtani, F.Y.; Alattas, S.H.; Almangour, T.A.; Aleanizy, F.S. Status of infectious disease content in the professional pharmacy curriculum in Saudi Arabia: Results of a national survey. *Saudi Pharm. J.* **2021**, *29*, 1492–1497. [CrossRef]

30. Jairoun, A.; Hassan, N.; Ali, A.; Jairoun, O.; Shahwan, M. Knowledge, attitude and practice of antibiotic use among university students: A cross sectional study in UAE. *BMC Public Health* **2019**, *19*, 518. [CrossRef]
31. Al-Taani, G.M.; Karasneh, R.A.; Al-Azzam, S.; Bin Shaman, M.; Jirjees, F.; Al-Obaidi, H.; Conway, B.R.; Aldeyab, M.A. Knowledge, Attitude, and Behavior about Antimicrobial Use and Resistance among Medical, Nursing and Pharmacy Students in Jordan: A Cross Sectional Study. *Antibiotics* **2022**, *11*, 1559. [CrossRef]
32. Molina-Romera, G.; Vazquez-Cancela, O.; Vazquez-Lago, J.M.; Montes-Villalba, R.A.; Roque, F.; Herdeiro, M.T.; Figueiras, A. Knowledge, Attitudes and Practice Regarding Antibiotic Prescription by Medical Interns: A Qualitative Study in Spain. *Antibiotics* **2023**, *12*, 457. [CrossRef]

healthcare

MDPI

Article

Evaluation of Outreach of Community Pharmacists in Public Health Services in Al-Jouf Region of Saudi Arabia: Findings and Implications

Abdulaziz Ibrahim Alzarea [1,*], Yusra Habib Khan [1], Abdullah Salah Alanazi [1,2], Nasser Hadal Alotaibi [1], Sami I. Alzarea [3], Ziyad Saeed Almalki [4], Saad S. Alqahtani [5] and Tauqeer Hussain Mallhi [1,2,*]

1 Department of Clinical Pharmacy, College of Pharmacy, Jouf University, Sakaka 72388, Saudi Arabia; yhkhan@ju.edu.sa (Y.H.K.); asdalananzi@ju.edu.sa (A.S.A.); nhalotaibi@ju.edu.sa (N.H.A.)
2 Health Sciences Research Unit, Jouf University, Sakaka 72388, Saudi Arabia
3 Department of Pharmacology, College of Pharmacy, Jouf University, Sakaka 72388, Saudi Arabia; samisz@ju.edu.sa
4 Department of Clinical Pharmacy, College of Pharmacy, Prince Sattam Bin Abdulaziz University, Al-Kharj 11942, Saudi Arabia; z.almalki@psau.edu.sa
5 Department of Clinical Pharmacy, College of Pharmacy, King Khalid University, Abha 62529, Saudi Arabia; ssalqahtani@jazanu.edu.sa
* Correspondence: aizarea@ju.edu.sa (A.I.A.); thhussain@ju.edu.sa (T.H.M.)

Abstract: Background: Diversifying the conventional role of community pharmacists from dispensing to involvement in public health services could help in optimized patient care and ultimately good health practices. The current study aimed to ascertain the involvement of community pharmacists, barriers to involvement, their preparedness towards the provision of public health services in the future, and effective strategies to improve their existing role, especially in remote areas of the Kingdom of Saudi Arabia. Methods: A cross-sectional study was conducted in the Al-Jouf region of Saudi Arabia (KSA), between January to April 2023. A convenient sampling technique was used to recruit community pharmacists (CPs). A self-designed and validated questionnaire was used for data collection. The relative importance index (RII) was utilized to rank the barriers to participation in public health services. Data were subjected to statistical analysis using SPSS. Results: This study recruited 119 participants (mean age: 32.2 ± 7.9; male gender: 67.2%). Of these, 91.6% were involved in the provision of public health services at community pharmacies. Majority of CPs (n = 114/119, 95.8%) provided drug use-related written information to the patients, and the least practiced service was screening of dyslipidemia (n = 81; 68.1%). According to RII, the major barrier was the lack of time given by patients (RII: 0.812). Overall, the majority of the pharmacists (n = 94/119; 79%) were willing to provide public health services. Most of the CPs reported that empowerment through education and awareness (n = 100/119; 84%) is most effective strategy to enhance the involvement of pharmacists in public health services. Conclusions: Findings of the present study underscored the adequate participation of community pharmacists in public health activities. Further studies are required in other remote regions of KSA to get a clear insight into the overall participation of community pharmacists in public health services and generalize the findings.

Keywords: community pharmacist; public health services; Al-Jouf; community pharmacies; health promotion; Saudi Arabia

check for updates

Citation: Alzarea, A.I.; Khan, Y.H.; Alanazi, A.S.; Alotaibi, N.H.; Alzarea, S.I.; Almalki, Z.S.; Alqahtani, S.S.; Mallhi, T.H. Evaluation of Outreach of Community Pharmacists in Public Health Services in Al-Jouf Region of Saudi Arabia: Findings and Implications. *Healthcare* **2023**, *11*, 2299. https://doi.org/10.3390/healthcare11162299

Academic Editor: Georges Adunlin

Received: 8 June 2023
Revised: 2 August 2023
Accepted: 8 August 2023
Published: 15 August 2023

1. Introduction

Apart from the conventional role of dispensing and compounding, pharmacist's role has evolved as a vital part of the multi-disciplinary workforce providing extended services at the community level [1,2]. However, this paradigm shift in pharmacist's role from dispensing to integrated involvement in public health services is pertinent, but limited to developed countries and needs further uplifting in other regions of the world [3]. These services at the community level include the provision of drug-related information, counseling regarding drug use, lifestyle modification, screening of chronic and infectious diseases, medication therapy management (MTM), drug interactions, potential and actual adverse drug reactions (ADRs), and awareness regarding immunization [4,5]. However, Community Pharmacists (CPs) are acknowledged as the most accessible healthcare professionals in the Kingdom of Saudi Arabia (KSA) [6–9].

Despite recommendations from World Health Organization (WHO) on pharmacists role in providing patient-oriented services, the participation of CPs in public health activities needs to be further strengthened by the relevant authorities around the globe [2]. If these recommendations are implemented, health benefits will be optimized, and patients will also benefit from CPs' knowledge and skills [10]. The new pharmacy model Vision 2030 proposed by the Saudi government, envisaged the provision of ambulatory pharmaceutical care services through community pharmacies by expanding the role of CPs [11]. Further studies in different regions of KSA can ascertain the current practices and help with the road map to achieve this new model vision.

The Vision Saudi Arabia 2030 program, envisioning an effective and more integrated healthcare system, was launched by the government of KSA in 2016. Among the fundamental objectives of the programs to promote improved health services include facilitating access, quality, and efficiency of healthcare services, promoting health risk prevention, and reinforcing traffic safety [12]. Different strategical plans were devised by the Ministry of Health (MOH) to keep the program afloat and achieve its ultimate goal [13]. Keeping up with the strategies, a new pharmacy model for Vision 2030 in Saudi Arabia was also devised that was in line with the one, five, seven, and nine number strategies of the MOH plan [11]. The Saudi Vision 2030 program emphasizes public health services, and this program needs to be implemented in all of the KSA. To ensure the current status of this program, there is a need to assess the public health services provided in remote areas and barriers to ensure full coverage, other than only being implemented in big studies.

There is a scarcity of information regarding the involvement of CPs in public health services, all over KSA, and it is pertinent to ascertain their factual involvement, especially in remote regions like Al-Jouf. Present study aimed to bridge the literature gap and also answer the aforementioned research questions. Al-Jouf region was selected because it has limited access to healthcare facilities and healthcare professionals and is located in a remote region. The current study will provide an actual picture of the services in remote areas rather than taking into account the outcomes of studies in metropolitan cities reporting varying levels of CPs' participation and hence requiring further investigation [10]. The rationale of the study was to bridge the literature gap regarding the problem statement. Few studies have been conducted regarding the role of pharmacists in community services in Saudi Arabia. Although good knowledge and preparedness of CPs in Saudi are previously reported, however, these studies were conducted mainly in cosmopolitan cities such as Jeddah, Makkah, Riyadh, and Madinah [14].

The present study aimed to ascertain the practices conducted in Al-Jouf, which is a remote region and comparatively has limited healthcare facilities, less developed infrastructure, and a smaller number of pharmacists as compared to other large cities of the countries. Due to these circumstances, very few pharmacists are attracted to this area, which will definitely impact the quantity and quality of the services provided by community pharmacists in this region. Moreover, authors belong to the Al-Jouf region. This study will further provide an outlook on the services in which CPs are involved in such remote regions compared to studies carried out in larger cities with sufficient resources and access to health facilities. This study also intended to identify the barriers to the participation, preparedness, and willingness of CPs towards the provision of additional services in the future, and recommendation of effective strategies to further improve the involvement of CPs in public health activities in Al-Jouf. To the best of our knowledge, previously conducted studies in smaller areas did not report the preparedness of the CPs to participate in such activities at the public health level [10]. The findings of the current study will fill the gap in the current literature, will reflect the factual involvement of CPs in Al-Jouf, and will pertinently provide effective strategies to overcome the barriers and enhance the participation of pharmacists in public health activities.

2. Materials and Methods

2.1. Ethical Approval

Prior to the commencement of the survey, the study was approved by the Local Committee on Bioethics (LCBE) of Jouf University (Reference no.: 7-10-43). Description of the study and its purpose was provided at the beginning of the survey. Informed consent was obtained from all the participants and their anonymity was maintained.

2.2. Study Design and Settings

A cross-sectional study was conducted among community pharmacists working in Al-Jouf province, Saudi Arabia. Data were collected over a period of four months (January to April 2022). Al-Jouf is one of the 13 provinces of KSA, having an estimated population of 0.5 million [15]. It is a less-developed province in the northern region sharing its border with Jordan, in comparison to the metropolitan provinces. Being a remote region, there is limited access to healthcare facilities as well as healthcare professionals including pharmacists. Inclusion criteria for this current study include: (1) a qualified pharmacist working in a community pharmacy, (2) willing to participate in the survey, (3) either male or female gender, (4) employee or self-employed, and (5) able to write and understand Arabic and English. Those participants who did not fulfill the criteria were excluded from the study. The flow diagram of the present study is shown in Figure 1.

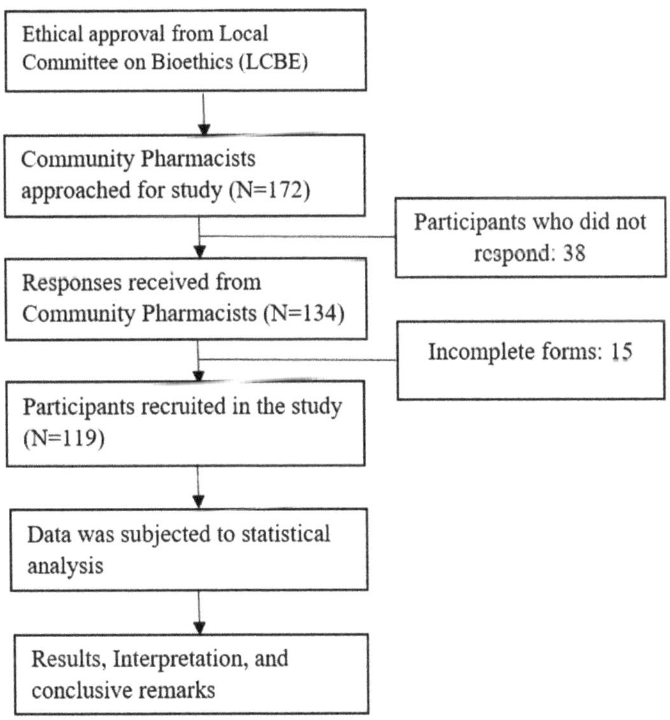

Figure 1. Study flow diagram.

2.3. Sampling Technique

A convenient sampling technique was used to collect the data from the three major cities of the Al-Jouf region, i.e., Sakaka, Dumat al-Jandal, and Qurayat. For data collection purposes, all the accessible pharmacies were identified and lists were prepared, regardless of the type of pharmacy (chain or single pharmacy). Investigators visited these community pharmacies in-person and collected data from the on-duty pharmacists. Data was collected on a paper-based study tool from those who consented to participate. Pharmacists who consented and were on duty were recruited in the survey by the investigators, ensuring to maintain anonymity.

2.4. Study Instrument

The data collection tool was self-designed with a literature review and consisted of close-ended questions [10,16–18]. The questionnaire was in English and Arabic, keeping in view the multi-cultural participants of KSA working at the community level and their better command of the language to avoid any inaccuracy. The questionnaire was reviewed by a panel of experts from different health professions for its content validity. After the content validity, recommended changes were made in the questionnaire before piloting. For face validity, and to assess comprehensibility, the study tool was pre-tested in a small sample (n = 30) for further clarity. Feedback from the CPs in the pilot study, not included in the final survey, was instilled into the final data collection tool. A Cronbach alpha value of 0.69 indicated the adequate reliability and consistency of the questionnaire.

The questionnaire consisted of five sections evaluating different aspects of CPs' involvement in public health services. Section I consisted of 10 questions related to the demographics of the study participants. Section II comprised of 17 close-ended questions assessing the involvement of CPs in different services in public health, classified under five different categories. Section III contained 14 questions assessing barriers to pharmacists' involvement in public health services on a 5-point Likert scale (1 = strongly agree, 2 = agree, 3 = neutral, 4 = disagree, and 5 = strongly disagree). The mean score and percentage of each item were used for further analysis. The score for each item was calculated to obtain the mean score, with 0 corresponding to the least and 5 to the highest score (range: 0–5). For this purpose, the Likert scale was reverse coded to get a maximum score as strongly agreed (5 = strongly agree, 4 = agree, 3 = neutral, 2 = disagree, and 1 = strongly disagree). Furthermore, percentage agreement was the cumulative frequency of responses of those who "strongly agree" and "agree" with the barriers. Moreover, "strongly disagree", "disagree", and "neutral" were interpreted as negative responses. Section IV consisted of six statements evaluating the preparedness of community pharmacists towards the provision of public health services on a similar 5-point Likert scale (1 = strongly agree to 5 = strongly disagree). Furthermore, the *positive attitude* of pharmacists towards role enhancement in public health services was indicated by *percentage agreement*, with the cumulative frequency and percentages of those with "strongly agree" and "agree", whereas, the *negative attitude* was depicted as "strongly disagree", "disagree", and "neutral". For scoring purposes, reverse coding was performed to get the maximum score correlating with an excellent level of willingness. The score range for willingness was 1–5, i.e., 1 = unwillingness, 2 = poor willingness, 3 = average willingness, 4 = good willingness, and 5 = excellent level of willingness to participate in the future. Lastly, Section V had seven statements aimed to evaluate the opinion of community pharmacists on the effective strategies to enhance public health role on a similar 5-point Likert scale (1 = strongly agree to 5 = strongly disagree). Re-coding and scoring system in the present study was adapted from previously conducted research investigations [16,19].

2.5. Data Collection

The current study collected data by self-administration of the paper-based study tool. Data was scrutinized, converted to an Excel sheet, and subjected to further statistical analysis. All the responses were checked, and only completed responses were included. Incomplete responses were excluded from further analysis.

2.6. Statistical Analysis

Data analysis was performed using Statistical Package for the Social Sciences (SPSS) version 25. Descriptive data were summarized as frequency and percentages (%). Continuous data were expressed as Mean ± SD. The p-value of <0.05 was considered statistically significant. Chi-square/Fischer test was used to evaluate the association between the involvement of community pharmacists and demographics. Percentage agreement (%) to the statements assessing the participation of CPs in public health activities and barriers in the provision of these services, a 5-point Likert scale was converted to 2 points, i.e., "agree" and "strongly agree" was re-coded as "agreed" while "disagree", "strongly disagree", and "neutral" was converted to "disagreed". Furthermore, to ascertain the significance and rank of the perceived barriers, relative importance index (RII) was used for ranking the barriers. RII equation was used, in which W = weight given to each statement by participant (5 = strongly agreed to 1 strongly disagreed), A = highest weight, and N = total number of participants. The highest value of RII ($0 \leq \text{RII} \leq 1$) corresponded to the main barrier.

$$\text{RII} = \frac{\sum \text{W}}{(\text{A} * \text{N})}$$

3. Results

3.1. Characteristics of Study Participants

A total of 172 community pharmacists working in Al-Jouf province were approached for the survey. The response rate was more than half of the approached participants (n = 119/172; 69.2%). Of these 172 participants, 38 did not respond, and 15 questionnaires were incomplete and were excluded from the study. A total of 119 participants were included in the study. The mean age of the study participants was 32.2 ± 7.9 years. Most of the participants were males (n = 80/119, 67.2%), Saudi nationals (n = 79/119, 66.4%), having age 20–30 years (n = 65/119, 54.6%), had Bachelors in Pharmacy (B. Pharmacy) degree (n = 87/119, 73.1%), working as an employee (n = 96/119, 80.7%), in chain pharmacy setup (n = 87/119, 71.4%), resident pharmacists (n = 88/119, 73.9%), and had 1–5 years of work experience (n = 52/119, 43.7%). Detailed demographic features of the participants are shown in Table 1.

Table 1. Demographic characteristics of the study participants (N = 119).

Variables	Frequency (%)
Gender	
Male	80 (67.2)
Female	39 (32.8)
Age	
20–30 years	65 (54.6)
31–40 years	40 (33.6)
>40 years	14 (11.8)
Nationality	
Saudi	79 (66.4)
Non-Saudi	40 (33.6)
Qualification	
Bachelors in Pharmacy	87 (73.1)
Doctor of Pharmacy	23 (19.3)
MPhil/MS	6 (5)
Ph.D.	3 (2.5)

Table 1. *Cont.*

Variables	Frequency (%)
Level of training	
Resident (Pharmacist)	88 (73.9)
Associated Consultant (Senior Pharmacist)	13 (10.9)
Consultant	18 (15.1)
Work experience	
≤5 years	59 (49.6)
6–10 years	37 (31.1)
11–15 years	13 (10.9)
>15 years	10 (8.4)
Type of community pharmacy	
Chain Pharmacy	85 (71.4)
Independent pharmacy	34 (28.6)
Average prescriptions filled per day	
<50	62 (52.1)
51–100	30 (25.2)
>100	27 (22.7)
Pharmacy ownership	
Employee	96 (80.7)
Owner	23 (19.3)

3.2. *Involvement of Community Pharmacists in Public Health Services*

The current study broadly categorized CPs' participation into five major categories, i.e., lifestyle modification, screening services, awareness and counseling, drug-related information, and miscellaneous public health services. A total of 17 public health services were classified under the aforementioned categories, in Table 2, assessing the involvement of community pharmacists in public health services. The most practiced public health service in Al-Jouf was the provision of drug-related information, i.e., the provision of written information on drug use by pharmacists, whereas, the least practiced was the involvement in screening services.

The majority of the participants (n = 109/119, 91.6%) were aware of the public health services. Most of the participants were involved in at least one public health service (Table 2). Of 119 community pharmacists, majority were involved in providing drug use-related information (n = 114/119, 95.8%), counseling patients while dispensing medications (n = 108/119, 90.8%), referral of patients to government hospitals (n = 98/119, 82.4%), and creating awareness and counseling regarding vaccination/immunization (n = 96/119, 80.7%). Additionally, many CPs were involved in lifestyle modification and prevention of diseases such as screening for hypertension (n = 89/119, 74.8%) and weight management (n = 87/119, 73.1%). While the least (n = 87/119, 68.1%) were involved in screening for dyslipidemia, physical activity promotion (n = 81/119, 68.1%), and counseling of married couples while initiating treatment for sexually transmitted diseases (STDs) (n = 81/119, 68.1%).

Significant association of socio-demographic factors with public health services has been observed (Table 3). Identification of health-related risks in the community was practiced more by males (n = 56/91; 61.5%; *p*-value: 0.021) as compared to female pharmacists. The practice of certain public health services such as smoke cessation (n = 51/85; 60%; *p*-value: 0.027), healthy eating (n = 51/84; 60.7%; *p*-value: 0.026), screening for hypertension (n = 44/89; 49.4%; *p*-value: 0.024), and screening of infectious diseases (n = 41/82; 50%; *p*-value: 0.017) was more among young pharmacists between age 20–30 years. Saudi nationals were more involved in smoking cessation (n = 62/85; 72.9%; *p*-value = 0.020), immunization (n = 68/96; 70.8%; *p*-value: 0.049), counseling regarding contraception and ECP pills (n = 68/94; 72.3; *p*-value: 0.016), and the identification of health-related risks in the community (n = 67/91; 73.6%; *p*-value: 0.005). Participants with bachelor degrees tended to be more involved in smoke cessation (n = 64/85; 75.3%; *p*-value: 0.023) as compared to those pharmacists with higher degrees. Work experience of an average of 1–5 years (n = 39/82, 47.6%; *p*-value = 0.013) was found to be associated with screening of infectious diseases. Moreover, CPs working in chain pharmacies were significantly associated with screening for hypertension (n = 58/89, 65.2%; *p*-value = 0.010). Those who were employees in community pharmacies were more involved in screening of infectious diseases (n = 60/82; 73.2%; *p*-value: 0.002), counseling regarding STDs (n = 60/81; 74.1; *p*-value: 0.007), promoting AMSP (n = 59/82; 72%; *p*-value < 0.001), identification of health-related risks in the community (n = 69/91; 75.8%; *p*-value: 0.014), and referral to a government hospital (n = 75/98; 76.5%; *p*-value: 0.012) as compared to those pharmacists who owned pharmacies. The CPs filling less prescriptions (<50 per day) were significantly involved in smoke cessation (*p*-value: 0.038), physical activity promotion (0.005), and counseling while dispensing medication (n = 52/108; 48.1%; *p*-value: 0.023).

Table 2. The extent of involvement of community pharmacists in public health services (N = 119).

Public Health Services	Yes n (%) *	No n (%)
Lifestyle modification		
Weight management	87 (73.1)	32 (26.9)
Smoking cessation	85 (71.4)	34 (28.6)
Physical activity promotion	81 (68.1)	38 (31.9)
Healthy eating	84 (70.6)	35 (29.4)
Screening services		
Screening for diabetes	83 (69.7)	36 (30.3)
Screening for hypertension	89 (74.8)	30 (25.2)
Screening for dyslipidemia	81 (68.1)	38 (31.9)
Screening of infectious diseases	82 (68.9)	37 (31.1)
Awareness and counseling		
Vaccination and immunization	96 (80.7)	23 (19.3)
Counseling regarding treatment for sexually transmitted diseases (STDs)	81 (68.1)	38 (31.9)
Counseling on emergency and other contraception pills	94 (79)	25 (21)
Drug-related information		
Counseling while dispensing medications	108 (90.8)	11 (9.2)
Providing written information on drug use	114 (95.8)	5 (4.2)
Personalized follow-up or private consultation	92 (77.3)	27 (22.7)
Promote antimicrobial stewardship programs	82 (68.9)	37 (31.1)
Miscellaneous Public Health Services		
Assessment to identify the health-related risks in community	91 (76.5)	28 (23.5)
Referral to government hospital	98 (82.4)	21 (17.6)

* n = frequency.

Table 3. Association of public health services with the demographics among community pharmacists.

Public Health Service	Gender	Age	Nationality	Qualification	Level of Training	Work Experience	Type of Community Pharmacy	Ownership of Pharmacy	Prescriptions Filled per Day
Weight management	0.379	0.113	0.081	0.150	0.120	0.535	0.069	0.610	0.200
Smoking cessation	0.086	**0.027**	**0.020**	**0.023**	0.387	0.062	0.654	0.802	**0.038**
Physical activity promotion	0.676	0.095	0.097	0.811	0.613	0.243	0.892	0.217	**0.005**
Healthy eating	0.085	**0.026**	0.203	0.231	0.178	0.068	0.081	1.000	0.252
Screening for diabetes	0.673	0.223	0.291	0.340	0.154	0.745	0.381	0.206	0.292
Screening for hypertension	1.000	**0.024**	0.117	0.169	0.629	0.959	**0.010**	0.059	0.917
Screening for dyslipidaemia	0.302	0.053	0.407	0.056	0.670	0.954	1.000	0.322	0.234
Screening of infectious diseases	0.095	**0.017**	0.063	0.573	0.137	**0.013**	0.051	**0.002**	0.750
Vaccination and immunisation	0.322	0.531	**0.049**	0.744	0.261	0.183	0.212	0.239	0.171
Counseling regarding STDs treatment	0.676	0.514	0.097	0.293	0.330	0.210	0.278	**0.007**	0.953
Counseling on ECP and other contraception pills	0.154	0.259	**0.016**	0.266	0.738	0.121	0.330	0.154	0.796
Counseling while dispensing medications	0.337	0.245	0.504	0.164	0.944	0.211	0.727	0.220	**0.023**
Providing written information on drug use	1.000	0.753	0.333	0.934	0.188	0.651	0.320	1.000	0.640
Personalized follow-up or private consultation	0.102	0.717	0.246	0.592	0.849	0.346	0.231	0.097	0.565
Promote AMSP	0.212	0.052	**0.023**	0.679	0.797	0.486	0.051	**<0.001**	0.641
Identification of the health-related risks in community	**0.021**	0.367	**0.005**	0.444	0.717	0.081	0231	**0.014**	0.332
Referral to government hospital	0.201	0.222	0.202	0.567	0.162	0.422	1.000	**0.012**	0.526

The table shows the *p*-value obtained from the chi-square test; *p*-value of less than 0.05 is considered statistically significant and is represented in bold, STD: Sexually transmitted diseases, ECP: Emergency contraceptive pill, AMSP: Antimicrobial stewardship programs.

Overall, pharmacists of male gender, of 20–30 years of age, majorly Saudi nationals, having a bachelor of pharmacy degree and work experience of 1–5 years, working in chain pharmacies as employees, and filling <50 prescriptions per day were significantly involved in the provision of public health services.

On the contrary, the training level of CPs was not linked with any public health service. In other words, the public health services such as weight management, screening of diabetes, screening for dyslipidemia, providing written information on drug use, and personalized follow-up or private consultation were not statistically linked with any demographic characteristic of CPs.

3.3. Barriers in Providing Public Health Services

Fourteen items were included in the present study that were potential barriers for pharmacists in delivering public health services (Table 4). All of the items in barriers reported mean scores greater than three. The highest ranked barrier reported that hindered CP's involvement in public health services was "*patients do not give time for such services*" (RI = 0.812; Mean score = 4.06 ± 0.85; 79%) followed by "*lack of coordination with other healthcare professionals*" (RI = 0.802; mean score = 4.01 ± 0.85; 76.5%), "*lack of access to training programs on public health*" (RI = 0.802; mean score = 4.01 ± 0.89; 75.6%), and "*shortage of pharmacy assistants or technicians*" (RI = 0.797; mean score = 3.98 ± 0.98; 78.2%). However, the lowest ranked barrier reported by CPs was a "*lack of confidence in my ability/level of information acquired by practicing pharmacists*" (RI: 0.748; mean score = 3.74 ± 1.15; 68.1%). The second lowest ranked barrier was "*patients generally have more urgent medical conditions*" (RI: 0.751; mean score = 3.76 ± 0.88; 68.9%). The third lowest ranked barriers were "*lack of financial compensation*" (RI: 0.761; mean score = 3.81 ± 1.00; 68.9%) and "*lack of patient demand for these services*" (RI: 0.761; mean score = 3.81 ± 0.91; 64.7%). The male gender tends to agree more with the barriers to involvement as compared to the female gender (Table 4); however, this gender association is not statistically significant. The association between the level of training of CPs with the perceived barriers was statistically significant. Resident pharmacists tend to agree that lack of clinical tools (n = 69/91; 75.8%; *p*-value: 0.041) and lack of coordination with other healthcare professionals (n = 667/91; 73.6%; *p*-value: 0.041) were the main barriers to the CPs involvement in public health services.

Table 4. Association of barriers in providing public health services with gender and level of training of community pharmacists (N = 119).

Barriers	Mean Score [a]	% Agreement [b] n (%)								RII [c]	Ranking [d]
		Total	Gender			Level of training of CP					
			Male	Female	*p*-Value *	RP	SP	C	*p*-Value **		
Lack of knowledge or clinical skills	3.87 ± 1.06	86 (72.3)	61 (70.9)	25 (29.1)	0.193	64 (74.4)	11 (12.8)	11 (12.8)	0.347	0.775	6
Shortage of time	3.93 ± 0.81	91 (76.5)	60 (65.9)	31 (34.1)	0.651	65 (71.4)	12 (13.2)	14 (15.4)	0.339	0.787	4
Shortage of pharmacists	3.88 ± 1.02	84 (70.6)	53 (63.1)	31 (36.9)	0.198	63 (75)	11 (13.1)	10 (11.9)	0.199	0.776	5
Shortage of pharmacy assistants or technicians	3.98 ± 0.98	93 (78.2)	62 (66.7)	31 (33.3)	1.000	70 (75.3)	11 (11.8)	12 (12.9)	0.405	0.797	3
Lack of confidence in my ability/level of information	3.74 ± 1.15	81 (68.1)	57 (70.4)	24 (29.6)	0.302	63 (77.8)	6 (7.4)	12 (14.8)	0.184	0.748	10
Patients do not give time for such services	4.06 ± 0.85	94 (79)	62 (66)	32 (34)	0.638	70 (74.5)	11 (11.7)	13 (13.8)	0.683	0.812	1
Lack of patient demand for these services	3.81 ± 0.91	77 (64.7)	54 (70.1)	23 (29.9)	0.416	55 (71.4)	11 (14.3)	11 (14.3)	0.280	0.761	8
Lack of financial compensation	3.8[illegible] ± 1.00	82 (68.9)	57 (69.5)	25 (30.5)	0.527	58 (70.7)	12 (14.6)	12 (14.6)	0.155	0.761	8
Lack of space in the pharmacy for such services	3.87 ± 0.95	84 (70.6)	57 (67.9)	27 (32.1)	0.833	63 (75)	11 (13.1)	10 (11.9)	0.199	0.773	7
Patients generally have more urgent medical conditions	3.76 ± 0.88	82 (68.9)	55 (67.1)	27 (32.9)	1.000	61 (74.4)	11 (13.4)	10 (12.2)	0.223	0.751	9
Legal and regulatory constraints/unclear regulatory environment	3.[illegible] ± 0.85	82 (68.9)	59 (72)	23 (28)	0.139	60 (73.2)	11 (13.4)	11 (13.4)	0.363	0.773	7
Lack of clinical tools	3.[illegible] ± 0.89	91 (76.5)	63 (69.2)	28 (30.8)	0.491	69 (75.8)	12 (13.2)	10 (11)	0.041	0.787	4
Lack of coordination with other healthcare professionals	4.0[illegible] ± 0.85	91 (76.5)	63 (69.2)	28 (30.8)	0.491	67 (73.6)	13 (14.3)	11 (12.1)	0.041	0.802	2
Lack of access to training programs on public health	4.[illegible] ± 0.89	90 (75.6)	61 (67.8)	29 (32.2)	0.823	69 (76.7)	11 (12.2)	10 (11.1)	0.087	0.802	2

CP: community pharmacist, RP: resident pharmacist, SP: senior pharmacist, C: consultant pharmacist, [a] Mean score ± SD on Likert scale: strongly disagree = 1; disagree = 2; neutral= 3; agree = 4; strongly agree = 5; SD: standard deviation; [b] Percentage agreement response is the summation of agree/strongly agree options, [c] RI: relative index, [d] Ranking according to the RII (0 ≤ RII ≤ 1)), * *p*-value obtained from chi-square test showing an association between barriers and genders; *p*-value < 0.05 is significant, ** *p*-value obtained from chi-square test showing an association between barriers and level of training of community pharmacists.

3.4. *Preparedness of Community Pharmacists towards Public Health Services*

The willingness of pharmacists to incorporate themselves into public health services was assessed using six statements. All of the items corresponding to the preparedness of CPs reported mean scores greater than four for the majority of the statements, indicating a good level of preparedness of CPs (Table 5). A higher proportion (79%) of participants reported a *positive attitude* by agreeing that *pharmacists in general are willing to provide public health services*, supplementing with the mean score of 4.19 ± 0.78, indicating a satisfactory level of preparedness. Association of gender with the preparedness of CPs' involvement was more in the male gender as compared to the females (Table 5); however, this gender association is not statistically significant. There was an association between the level of preparedness and level of training of CPs (*p*-value: 0.037). Resident pharmacist indicated higher levels of preparedness (n = 57/79; 72.2%) where majority of them agreed that their pharmacies are prepared to provide public health services.

Table 5. Preparedness of community pharmacists towards public health services and their association with gender and level of training of community pharmacists (N = 119).

Statement	Mean Score [a] (Mean ± SD)	Percentage Agreement [b] n (%)							*p*-Value **
		Total	Gender		*p*-Value *	Level of Training of CP			
			Male	Female		RP	SP	C	
I feel that I have enough clinical knowledge to provide public health services	4.07 ± 0.89	87 (73.1)	61 (70.1)	26 (29.9)	0.279	63 (72.4)	8 (9.2)	16 (18.4)	0.195
I feel that I have enough clinical experience to provide public health services	4.03 ± 0.78	91 (76.5)	64 (70.3)	27 (29.7)	0.250	66 (72.5)	9 (9.9)	16 (17.6)	0.363
My pharmacy is currently prepared to provide public health services	3.87 ± 0.93	79 (66.4)	55 (69.6)	24 (30.4)	0.536	57 (72.2)	6 (7.6)	16 (20.3)	0.037
I think pharmacists in general are willing to provide public health services	4.19 ± 0.78	94 (79)	64 (68.1)	30 (31.9)	0.811	68 (72.3)	10 (10.6)	16 (17)	0.535
I have sufficient references to provide public health services in daily practice	4.02 ± 0.94	90 (75.6)	60 (66.7)	30 (33.3)	1.000	65 (72.2)	9 (10)	16 (17.8)	0.340
I am satisfied with my role as community pharmacist	3.95 ± 1.01	86 (72.3)	57 (66.3)	29 (33.7)	0.829	59 (68.6)	12 (14)	15 (17.4)	0.086

CP: community pharmacist, RP: resident pharmacist, SP: senior pharmacist, C: consultant pharmacist, SD: standard deviation; [a] Mean score ± SD on Likert scale: strongly disagree = 1; disagree = 2; neutral = 3; agree = 4; strongly agree = 5; [b] Percentage agreement response is the summation of agree/strongly agree options; * *p*-value obtained from chi-square test showing an association between strategies and gender; *p*-value < 0.05 is significant; ** *p*-value obtained from chi-square test showing an association between strategies and level of training of community pharmacists.

3.5. *Strategies to Enhance the Public Health Role of Community Pharmacists*

There were seven proposed strategies to enhance the role of CPs in public health services (Table 6). The majority of the pharmacists agreed that *"empowerment through education and awareness"* (n = 100/119; 84%), *teaching the use of new technologies* (n = 99; 83.2%), and *teaching macro-level public health activities* (n = 99/119; 83.2%) will be the most effective techniques in improving the role of CPs in public health. The association of gender with strategies to improve CPs role was significant for the *teaching of macro-level public health activities* strategy, with the male gender agreeing more than the female gender (n = 71/99; 71.7%; *p*-value: 0.034). However, there is no significant association between the training level of CPs and their agreement to strategies for the enhancement of the future role of pharmacists.

Table 6. Strategies to enhance community pharmacists' involvement in public health services and their association with gender and level of training of community pharmacists.

Strategies to Improve CPs' Involvement in Public Health Services in Future	Percentage Agreement [a] n (%)							
	Total	Gender		p-Value *	Level of Training of CPs			p-Value **
		Male	Female		RP	SP	C	
Empowerment through education and awareness	100 (84)	67 (67)	33 (33)	1.000	72 (72)	10 (10)	18 (18)	0.121
Empowerment through direct remuneration of pharmacists	95 (79.8)	63 (66.3)	32 (33.7)	0.809	68 (71.6)	11 (11.6)	16 (16.8)	0.482
The use of new technologies and social media in practice	96 (80.7)	63 (65.6)	33 (34.4)	0.622	69 (71.9)	10 (10.4)	17 (17.7)	0.273
Teaching the use of new technologies	99 (83.2)	67 (67.7)	32 (32.3)	0.800	73 (73.7)	10 (10.1)	16 (16.2)	0.675
Encouraging collaboration between pharmacists and other healthcare professionals	97 (81.5)	68 (70.1)	29 (29.9)	0.209	72 (74.2)	9 (9.3)	16 (16.5)	0.376
Tackling a number of barriers	96 (80.7)	66 (68.8)	30 (31.3)	0.469	71 (74)	10 (10.4)	15 (15.6)	0.905
Teaching macro-level public health activities	99 (83.2)	71 (71.7)	28 (28.3)	0.034	74 (74.7)	10 (10.1)	15 (15.2)	0.812

CP: community pharmacist, RP: resident pharmacist, SP: senior pharmacist, C: consultant pharmacist, SD: standard deviation; [a] Responses of the participants who agreed and strongly agreed are included; * p-value obtained from chi-square test showing an association between gender with CPs' preparedness towards involvement in public health services; p-value < 0.05 is considered significant; ** p-value obtained from chi-square test showing an association between level of training and preparedness of CPs towards involvement in public health services.

4. Discussion

The current study is the first of its kind, assessing the outreach of community pharmacists in public health services in Al-Jouf, a remote region in Saudi Arabia with limited access to healthcare facilities. The findings of the present study documented that the majority of the registered pharmacists working in such remote vicinity had a good level of understanding of public health services. Overall, these findings reflect the shift from traditional compounding and dispensing services towards extended roles of community pharmacists in public health. These findings were in line with the studies conducted across the globe [2,20,21]. Previously conducted studies in Saudi Arabia also coincide with these findings [22]. However, there is a dearth of actual data from other remote regions, as the majority of the studies were from big cities. Additionally, this study evaluated the level and extent of preparedness of pharmacists to extend their roles in achieving the Saudi Vision 2030, not only in metropolitan cities but all over the country.

Interestingly, most of the pharmacists were aware of public health services in the current study. This adequate awareness of pharmacists regarding public health services at the community level corroborates with the findings of studies conducted in Pakistan, Scotland, and Nigeria reporting 99%, 90%, and 80% awareness, respectively [16,18,20,23]. Outcomes of the present study were more inclined toward CPs' role in the provision of drug use-related information, patient counseling while drug-dispensing, and creating awareness regarding vaccination. These are similar to other previously conducted studies in Malaysia and Pakistan [16,24]. On the contrary, it is pertinent to note that in developed nations, CPs were more likely involved in screening and lifestyle modification services, including screening of chronic diseases such as diabetes and hypertension [25–30]. Additionally, screening for dyslipidemia was considerably low in the present study but still did not corroborate with the studies conducted in Pakistan and Canada, in which extremely low (i.e., 4.8% and 6.5%, respectively) number of CPs were practicing dyslipidemia screening [16,31].

Despite the awareness of pharmacists in public health services, the majority were not involved in the provision of certain services, particularly in lifestyle modifications to prevent diseases and improve patient health outcomes. This lack of involvement is an indication that factors are hindering the provision of these services. To overcome these barriers, various strategies will need to optimize the outcome and further enhance CPs' role in public health services. The most eminent and highest-ranked barrier reported in this study indicated that patients have insufficient time to avail these services offered by the CPs, aligning with the results of the previous study [16]. Moreover, these findings highlight the fact that the highest ranked barrier is not due to the inefficiency of CPs, but due to the lack of time patients have to avail the expert opinion on drugs and health related issues of the pharmacists. This could also be due to unawareness of the general public about the significance and potential benefits of pharmacist-led counseling to achieve health goals. To eradicate this barrier, awareness campaigns and promotional techniques regarding counseling by pharmacists would immensely help the end-user. Our study also documented similar strategies to be the most effective, i.e., awareness and educational campaigns similar to those recommended in studies conducted in Australia, USA, and Pakistan [16,32,33].

The current study identified that there is insufficient communication with other healthcare professionals as the 2nd highest-ranked barrier. These findings are in agreement with the results of previously conducted studies in Indonesia, Canada, and Pakistan [16,34,35]. Promoting collaboration of pharmacists with other healthcare professionals via the introduction of mandatory training sessions and ward rounds (if working at hospital levels), via telecommunication (providing information about the nearby hospitals and clinics) to bridge the gap will help in eradicating this miscommunication. This strategy will eventually lead to improved patient care by integration of CPs in the system [16,33]. Another significant barrier was highlighted in the current study was lack of appropriate training programs that need to be organized to update the knowledge and skills of the pharmacists working in community setups. The similar results have been reported by other studies [16,34,35].

On-job training sessions, conferences, and online training sessions must be organized by pharmacist working in public and private sectors, keeping in mind the continuous recurrence of COVID pandemic waves. However, the present study reported a statistically significant association of resident pharmacists with the reporting of this barrier. This might indicate that at the residency level, resident pharmacists have limited or no access to healthcare professionals. For this reason, CPs must be trained and provided access to form liaisons with other healthcare workers. A interdisciplinary training program will also help to eradicate this barrier.

Less number of pharmacy assistants or pharmacy technicians was identified as third most reported barrier. This indicated that due to increased workload, CPs are unable to participate in public health services, and their role is limited to traditional services. These findings are in line with a survey conducted in Nigeria [36]. Contrarily, it does not coincide with a study conducted in Pakistan that does not recognize the shortage of technical staff [16]. These results necessitate a dire need to have pharmacy technicians according to the workload of the pharmacies. In this context, the health authorities can design framework to determine the number of pharmacy technicians required by a pharmacy in order to facilitate the pharmacists for public health services. This barrier is frequently reported by male and resident pharmacists in this study. However, this could be due to the higher number of male participants in our study.

Regarding the preparedness of CPs to get involved in provision of public health services, this study indicated a satisfactory level of willingness and positive attitude of CPs toward their involvement in public health services. These results corroborate with previous studies conducted in China, USA, Pakistan, and Nigeria [16,37–39] where CPs showed positive attitudes and preparedness for public health services. These findings reflected that CPs have adequate clinical experience which could be no obstacle in the provision of public health services, resonating with their competency. However, the resident pharmacists were significantly more inclined, and they were currently prepared to provide public health services. On the other hand, there was no statistically significant association between gender and level of preparedness for public health services.

Current study also evaluated plausible strategies that would enhance the involvement of CPs in public health services. Empowerment through education and awareness was the most recommended strategical technique recommended by the CPs. These recommendations are similar to other studies conducted in various parts of the world. Other popularly documented strategies by CPs included incorporating teaching and training sessions demonstrating the use of new technologies at macro-level public health activities, hence, extending and enhancing the role of community pharmacists. Interestingly, the female gender tends to be significantly associated with the encouragement of the introduction of new technologies at the macro level.

It is important to note that Saudi pharmacists were almost double in proportion as compared to non-Saudi pharmacists that might be a possible reason for efficient delivery of the public health services in this study. Previous studies have indicated that expats being unaccustomed with the culture and having language barrier are less involved in public health services. Contrary to the previous studies, current findings highlighted that a major proportion of the CPs were employees rather than self employed as compared to a previous survey in KSA where the majority were owners and hence more business-oriented than patient-centered [40]. However, it was consistent with the findings of a study conducted in Pakistan where 84.8% of pharmacists were working as employees [16]. These two factors could be linked to the difference in public health services provision to such an extent in a remote area such as Al-Jouf. Furthermore, it is pertinent to note that various other factors may limit and facilitate the provision of public health services in community pharmacies that are not ascertained by the current study such as lack of updated knowledge and skills, lack of recognition, trust on CP's knowledge and skills at the patient level, and inaccessibility to the medical records of patients.

4.1. Recommendations for Stakeholders

The fact is acknowledged that the Ministry of Health of Saudi Arabia is in the continuous process of updating the regulations regarding the provision of public health services at the community level [30]. However, to achieve the Saudi Vision 2030, implementation needs to be expedited. Pharmacists working at the community level must be well equipped in every aspect such as updated medical, pharmaceutical, and clinical knowledge, competitive skills, proper professional qualification, and good managerial skills to subdue perceived barriers with a proper sense of responsibility. However, currently, the Saudi health authorities have a paucity of working guidelines in place for community pharmacists to diligently carry out their recommended duties [41]. Hence, there is a dire need at the policy making and implementation level. The policymakers such as the Ministry of Health, Saudi Food and Drug Authority (SFDA), Saudi Pharmaceutical Society (SPS), Saudi Patient Safety Center (SPSC), and other Pharmacists associations in the country should collaborate and achieve the standard operating procedures (SOPs) being practiced worldwide [42–44]. Continued medical education, periodic training sessions, and refresher on-job courses must be designed, conducted, and made mandatory for practicing by relevant professional organizations to help the CPs remain up-to-date and efficient in performing their roles [30,45,46]. If implemented at national level, CPs services will be standardized and eventually will help to achieve the Saudi Vision 2030 efficiently. These findings also encourage global pharmacist organizations to focus on extended roles of CPs. Pharmacists led public health services should be integrated into pharmacy curriculum and residency programs. There is a need of collaboration between public health and pharmacy organizations at global level.

4.2. Limitations and Strengths of the Study

The present study is limited by a smaller sample size due to the limited pharmacies in Al-Jouf, which could be a potential bias, followed by the COVID pandemic still being present and possibly fewer pharmacists working at the time of data collection. Additionally, there is a strong probability that the pharmacists who participated in the study could be different and respond differently from those who did not participate, i.e., as only pharmacists in Al-Jouf pharmacies were approached. Moreover, a convenient sampling technique was used for data collection, which limits the generalizability of the findings. Furthermore, even though the association between the variables might exist, due to the cross sectional study design, we were unable to establish causal inferences. This study was conducted in a single region and might not be extrapolated to other regions having varying CPs' practicing cultures. Additionally, the recruited participants may have the bias of being part of the population who was less inclined to participate in such activities. Nevertheless, this study is strengthened by being the first representation of the estimation of CPs' participation in public health services in the Al-Jouf region in Saudi Arabia. Furthermore, previous studies did not compile and discuss data of both Saudi nationals and non-Saudi nationals, which is another strength of this survey.

4.3. Implications of the Current Study for Practice

The motivators to improve the participation of CPs in public health services might include incentives and rewards, which could be vital for the shift towards patient-oriented practice at the community pharmacy level [47]. Furthermore, there is a need to conduct qualitative analysis in the future to better evaluate the specific factors influencing the participation of community pharmacists towards public health services, both barriers and facilitators. Specifically, the current study will improve health outcomes by enhancing CPs' role in remote regions with meager health services and restricted access to them, such as Al-Jouf. Making strategies to overcome these barriers is the utmost need of the hour and the responsibility of concerned health authorities to substantiate the role of pharmacists working in community pharmacies regarding participation in public health services. Furthermore, the findings of this study can be contemplated for various similar regions like Al-Jouf. These outcomes will also help in increasing general clinical pharmacy services and specialized ambulatory care services [11].

5. Conclusions

The present study underscored the adequate involvement of pharmacists in public health services in remote regions of the KSA. Study recruits reflected a higher and satisfactory inclination towards future participation in current and expanding practices. Additionally, continued education will prove to be beneficial in further involvement of pharmacists in the activities in which they were less likely to be involved currently. Furthermore, pharmacists should self-participate and play a proactive role for the betterment of their profession and enhancement of their role. Moreover, further studies will be required to evaluate the outcomes of the recommended strategies provided in the current study to further enhance the role of community pharmacists. Finally, policies should be in place and strategies to implement these policies and integrate pharmacists in more clinical and public health roles should be expedited by the relevant health authorities.

Author Contributions: Conceptualization, A.I.A., Y.H.K. and T.H.M.; Data curation, A.S.A., N.H.A., S.I.A. and A.I.A.; Formal analysis, T.H.M., A.I.A. and Z.S.A.; Funding acquisition, A.I.A.; Investigation, A.I.A., Y.H.K., S.I.A., S.S.A. and N.H.A.; Methodology, Y.H.K., Z.S.A., A.S.A. and T.H.M.; Project administration, A.I.A. and T.H.M.; Software, A.S.A. and N.H.A.; Supervision, Y.H.K. and A.I.A.; Validation, S.I.A., S.S.A. and T.H.M.; Visualization, A.S.A. and A.I.A.; Writing—original draft, A.I.A., T.H.M., Y.H.K. and N.H.A.; Writing—review and editing, S.I.A., Z.S.A. and S.S.A. All authors have read and agreed to the published version of the manuscript.

Funding: This work was funded by the Prince Nawwaf bin Abdelaziz Chair for Sustainable Development in collaboration with the Deanship of Scientific Research at Jouf University under grant No. DSR2021-Prince Nawaf bin Abdulaziz Chair-04.

Institutional Review Board Statement: Prior to the commencement of the survey, the study was approved by the Local Committee on Bioethics (LCBE) of Jouf University (Reference no.: 7-10-43).

Informed Consent Statement: Informed consent was obtained from all subjects involved in the study.

Data Availability Statement: All underlying data are presented in this manuscript.

Acknowledgments: The authors gratefully acknowledged the financial support from Prince Nawwaf bin Abdelaziz Chair for Sustainable Development in collaboration with the Deanship of Scientific Research at Jouf University under grant No. DSR2021-Prince Nawaf bin Abdulaziz Chair-04.

Conflicts of Interest: The authors declare no conflict of interest.

References

1. Bouvy, M.L. *Integrating Pharmacy Services in Primary Care*; Oxford University Press: Oxford, UK, 2014; Volume 22, pp. 373–374.
2. Van Lerberghe, W. *The World Health Report 2008: Primary Health Care: Now More Than Ever*; World Health Organization: Geneva, Switzerland, 2008.
3. Twigg, M.J.; Wright, D.; Kirkdale, C.L.; Desborough, J.A.; Thornley, T. The UK pharmacy care plan service: Description, recruitment and initial views on a new community pharmacy intervention. *PLoS ONE* **2017**, *12*, e0174500.
4. Thananithisak, C.; Nimpitakpong, P.; Chaiyakunapruk, N. Activities and perceptions of pharmacists providing tobacco control services in community pharmacy in Thailand. *Nicotine Tob. Res.* **2008**, *10*, 921–925. [CrossRef] [PubMed]
5. Gillani, S.W.; Rahman, S.A.U.; Mohammad Abdul, M.I.; Sulaiman, S.A.S. Assessment of community pharmacists' perceptions of healthcare services in Saudi Arabia. *J. Pharm. Health Serv. Res.* **2017**, *8*, 269–274. [CrossRef]
6. Al-Arifi, M.N. Patients' perception, views and satisfaction with pharmacists' role as health care provider in community pharmacy setting at Riyadh, Saudi Arabia. *Saudi Pharm. J.* **2012**, *20*, 323–330. [CrossRef]
7. Al-Jedai, A.; Qaisi, S.; Al-Meman, A. Pharmacy practice and the health care system in Saudi Arabia. *Can. J. Hosp. Pharm.* **2016**, *69*, 231. [CrossRef] [PubMed]
8. Al-Tannir, M.; Alharbi, A.I.; Alfawaz, A.S.; Zahran, R.I.; AlTannir, M. Saudi adults satisfaction with community pharmacy services. *Springerplus* **2016**, *5*, 774. [CrossRef] [PubMed]

9. Alhaddad, M.S. Youth experience with community pharmacy services and their perceptions toward implementation of medication therapy management services by community pharmacists in the Western Region of Saudi Arabia. *Ther. Innov. Regul. Sci.* **2019**, *53*, 95–99. [CrossRef]
10. Almanasef, M.; Almaghaslah, D.; Kandasamy, G.; Vasudevan, R.; Batool, S. Involvement of community pharmacists in public health services in Asir Region, Saudi Arabia: A cross-sectional study. *Int. J. Clin. Pract.* **2021**, *75*, e14940. [CrossRef]
11. Alomi, Y.A. New pharmacy model for vision 2030 in Saudi Arabia. *J. Pharm. Pract. Community Med.* **2017**, *3*, 194–196. [CrossRef]
12. Saudi Vision 2030. Available online: https://www.vision2030.gov.sa/v2030/vrps/hstp/ (accessed on 3 June 2023).
13. National Transformation Program 2020. Available online: http://www.vision2030.gov.sa/en/ntp (accessed on 3 June 2023).
14. Hämmerlein, A.; Griese, N.; Schulz, M. Medication safety: Survey of drug-related problems identified by community pharmacies. *Ann. Pharmacother.* **2007**, *41*, 1825–1832. [CrossRef]
15. Atlas, W.D. World Data Atlas—Saudi Arabia. Available online: https://knoema.com/atlas/Saudi-Arabia/Al-Jouf (accessed on 6 June 2023).
16. Ijaz, E.; Amin, F.; Khan, Y.H.; Alanazi, A.S.; Mallhi, T.H.; Alzarea, A.I.; Salman, M.; Alotaibi, N.H. Ascertaining the Outreach of Community Pharmacist's Interventions in Public Health and Extended Pharmacy Services: A Cross Sectional Analysis. *Lat. Am. J. Pharm.* **2022**, *41*, 1398–1407.
17. Erku, D.A.; Mersha, A.G. Involvement of community pharmacists in public health priorities: A multi-center descriptive survey in Ethiopia. *PLoS ONE* **2017**, *12*, e0180943.
18. Rogers, C.J.; Bahr, K.O.; Benjamin, S.M. Attitudes and barriers associated with seasonal influenza vaccination uptake among public health students; a cross-sectional study. *BMC Public Health* **2018**, *18*, 1–8.
19. Mallhi, T.H.; Khan, Y.H.; Tanveer, N.; Bukhsh, A.; Khan, A.H.; Aftab, R.A.; Khan, O.H.; Khan, T.M. Awareness and knowledge of Chikungunya infection following its outbreak in Pakistan among health care students and professionals: A nationwide survey. *PeerJ* **2018**, *6*, e5481. [PubMed]
20. Rosenthal, M.M.; Breault, R.R.; Austin, Z.; Tsuyuki, R.T. Pharmacists' self-perception of their professional role: Insights into community pharmacy culture. *J. Am. Pharm. Assoc.* **2011**, *51*, 363–367, 368a.
21. Javeed, A.; Mahmood, K.T. Community pharmacy practice in Pakistan: From past to present-a review. *J. Pharm. Sci. Res.* **2012**, *4*, 1703.
22. Rayes, I.K.; Hassali, M.A.; Abduelkarem, A.R. The role of pharmacists in developing countries: The current scenario in the United Arab Emirates. *Saudi Pharm. J.* **2015**, *23*, 470–474.
23. Pfleger, D.E.; McHattie, L.W.; Diack, H.L.; McCaig, D.J.; Stewart, D.C. Views, attitudes and self-assessed training needs of Scottish community pharmacists to public health practice and competence. *Pharm. World Sci.* **2008**, *30*, 801–809. [CrossRef]
24. Kho, B.P.; Hassali, M.A.; Lim, C.J.; Saleem, F. Challenges in the management of community pharmacies in Malaysia. *Pharm. Pract.* **2017**, *15*. [CrossRef]
25. Paluck, E.C.; Stratton, T.P.; Eni, G.O. Community pharmacists' participation in health education and disease prevention activities. *Can. J. Public Health Rev. Can. De Sante Publique* **1994**, *85*, 389–392.
26. Eades, C.E.; Ferguson, J.S.; O'Carroll, R.E. Public health in community pharmacy: A systematic review of pharmacist and consumer views. *BMC Public Health* **2011**, *11*, 582. [CrossRef]
27. Scott, D.M.; Strand, M.; Undem, T.; Anderson, G.; Clarens, A.; Liu, X. Assessment of pharmacists' delivery of public health services in rural and urban areas in Iowa and North Dakota. *Pharm. Pract.* **2016**, *14*. [CrossRef] [PubMed]
28. Alhomoud, F.K.; Kunbus, A.; Ameer, A.; Alhomoud, F. Quality Assessment of community pharmacy services provided in the United Arab Emirates: Patient experience and satisfaction. *J. Appl. Pharm. Sci.* **2016**, *6*, 17–23.
29. Alkhamis, A. Health care system in Saudi Arabia: An overview. *East. Mediterr. Health J.* **2012**, *18*, 1078–1080. [CrossRef]
30. Rasheed, M.K.; Alqasoumi, A.; Hasan, S.S.; Babar, Z.-U.-D. The community pharmacy practice change towards patient-centered care in Saudi Arabia: A qualitative perspective. *J. Pharm. Policy Pract.* **2020**, *13*, 59. [CrossRef]
31. Laliberté, M.-C.; Perreault, S.; Damestoy, N.; Lalonde, L. Ideal and actual involvement of community pharmacists in health promotion and prevention: A cross-sectional study in Quebec, Canada. *BMC Public Health* **2012**, *12*, 192. [CrossRef] [PubMed]
32. Roberts, A.S.; Benrimoj, S.I.C.; Chen, T.F.; Williams, K.A.; Hopp, T.R.; Aslani, P. Understanding practice change in community pharmacy: A qualitative study in Australia. *Res. Soc. Adm. Pharm.* **2005**, *1*, 546–564. [CrossRef]
33. Agomo, C.O.; Ogunleye, J.; Portlock, J. Enhancing the public health role of community pharmacists—A qualitative research utilising the theoretical domains framework. *Innov. Pharm.* **2020**, *11*. [CrossRef]
34. Puspitasari, H.P.; Faturrohmah, A.; Hermansyah, A. Do Indonesian community pharmacy workers respond to antibiotics requests appropriately? *Trop. Med. Int. Health* **2011**, *16*, 840–846. [CrossRef]
35. Wong, L. *Ontario Pharmacy Smoking Cessation Program: A Descriptive Analysis, 2011–2016*; University of Toronto: Toronto, ON, Canada, 2019.
36. Osemene, K.P.; Erhun, W.O. Evaluation of community pharmacists' involvement in public health activities in Nigeria. *Braz. J. Pharm. Sci.* **2018**, *54*. [CrossRef]
37. Fang, Y.; Yang, S.; Feng, B.; Ni, Y.; Zhang, K. Pharmacists' perception of pharmaceutical care in community pharmacy: A questionnaire survey in Northwest China. *Health Soc. Care Community* **2011**, *19*, 189–197.
38. Kotecki, J.E.; Elanjian, S.I.; Torabi, M.R. Health promotion beliefs and practices among pharmacists. *J. Am. Pharm. Assoc.* **2000**, *40*, 773–779. [CrossRef]

39. Oparah, A.C.; Okojie, O.O. Health promotion perceptions among community pharmacists in Nigeria. *Int. J. Pharm. Pract.* **2005** *13*, 213–221. [CrossRef]
40. Dunlop, J.A.; Shaw, J.P. Community pharmacists' perspectives on pharmaceutical care implementation in New Zealand. *Pharm World Sci.* **2002**, *24*, 224–230. [CrossRef] [PubMed]
41. Erah, P.O.; Nwazuoke, J.C. Identification of standards for pharmaceutical care in Benin City. *Trop. J. Pharm. Res.* **2002**, *1*, 55–66. [CrossRef]
42. Centre SPSC. Saudi Patient Safety Centre. 2019. Available online: https://www.spsc.gov.sa/English/Pages/Home.aspx (accessed on 3 June 2023).
43. The Saudi Pharmaceutical Society (SPS). 2019. Available online: https://www.sipha-sps.com/about-us (accessed on 3 June 2023).
44. Authority SFaD. Saudi Food and Drug Authority. 2019. Available online: https://www.sfda.gov.sa/en (accessed on 3 June 2023).
45. Al-Arifi, M.N.; Al-Dhuwaili, A.A.; Gubara, O.A.; Al-Omar, H.A.; Al-Sultan, M.S.; Saeed, R.I.M. Pharmacists' understanding and attitudes towards pharmaceutical care in Saudi Arabia. *Saudi Pharm. J.* **2007**, *15*, 146–159.
46. Ishita, D.K.; Dureja, H. Role of community pharmacist in ensuring better healthcare. *Chron. Pharmabiz* **2004**, *4*, 29.
47. Amsler, M.R.; Murray, M.D.; Tierney, W.M.; Brewer, N.; Harris, L.E.; Marrero, D.G.; Weinberger, M. Pharmaceutical care in chain pharmacies: Beliefs and attitudes of pharmacists and patients. *J. Am. Pharm. Assoc.* **2001**, *41*, 850–855. [CrossRef]

healthcare MDPI

Review

The State of Pharmacoeconomics Education in the Doctor of Pharmacy Curriculum amid the Changing Face of Pharmacy Practice

Georges Adunlin [1,*], Jordan Skiera [2], Chandler S. Cupp [2], Askal Ayalew Ali [3] and Serge Amani Yao Afeli [4]

1 Department of Pharmaceutical, Social and Administrative Sciences, McWhorter School of Pharmacy, Samford University, Birmingham, AL 35229, USA
2 McWhorter School of Pharmacy, Samford University, Birmingham, AL 35229, USA; jskiera@samford.edu (J.S.); ccupp@samford.edu (C.S.C.)
3 Economic, Social and Administrative Pharmacy (ESAP), College of Pharmacy and Pharmaceutical Sciences, Institute of Public Health, Florida A&M University, Tallahassee, FL 323107, USA; askal.ali@famu.edu
4 Department of Pharmaceutical and Administrative Sciences, Presbyterian College School of Pharmacy, Clinton, SC 29325, USA; safeli@presby.edu
* Correspondence: gadunlin@samford.edu

Abstract: (1) Background: Continuous growth in pharmaceutical expenditure indicates the need for more advanced pharmacoeconomics evaluations to optimize healthcare outcomes and resource allocation. This study assesses the extent to which accredited pharmacy colleges in the United States cover pharmacoeconomics content within the didactic curriculum of their Doctor of Pharmacy (PharmD) programs. (2) Methods: We conducted a systematic search of the websites of accredited professional-degree programs in pharmacy schools located in the United States to identify pertinent content related to pharmacoeconomics. (3) Results: Out of 141 pharmacy programs, a total of 111 programs of varying sizes were found to have publicly accessible information regarding the content of their pharmacoeconomic curricula on their websites. All these programs required the inclusion of pharmacoeconomics content in their curricula. An examination of course syllabi revealed that the goals and descriptions were broad, aiming to provide students with an introductory understanding of the principles of pharmacoeconomics. The number of credit hours allocated to pharmacoeconomics education ranged from one to seven across the programs. The approach to delivering pharmacoeconomics content varied among the programs. (4) Conclusions: Advanced knowledge of the principles of pharmacoeconomics must be an integral component of all PharmD curricula to prepare pharmacists to assess the rational use of pharmacy products and services, improve clinical outcomes, and mitigate healthcare expenditures.

Keywords: pharmacoeconomics; pharmacy education; teaching; health outcomes research; United States

Citation: Adunlin, G.; Skiera, J.; Cupp, C.S.; Ali, A.A.; Afeli, S.A.Y. The State of Pharmacoeconomics Education in the Doctor of Pharmacy Curriculum amid the Changing Face of Pharmacy Practice. *Healthcare* **2023**, *11*, 2923. https://doi.org/10.3390/healthcare11222923

Academic Editor: Luk Hsiang Ning

Received: 25 September 2023
Revised: 30 October 2023
Accepted: 2 November 2023
Published: 8 November 2023

1. Introduction

Pharmacoeconomics is a sub-discipline of health economics that focuses on the economic evaluation of pharmaceutical products, treatments, and healthcare interventions [1]. It involves the application of economic principles and methods to assess the value, efficiency, and outcomes associated with various healthcare interventions, particularly in the context of pharmaceuticals [2].

The major topics involved in pharmacoeconomics include cost-effectiveness, cost-minimization, cost-utility, and cost-benefit analyses. It was not until the emergence of "evidence-based" medicine that notable advances were achieved in the use of pharmacoeconomics to identify, measure, and compare the costs and consequences of pharmaceutical products and services. Advances in new technologies have led to an exponential increase in competing treatments for a wide range of diseases [3,4]. Consequently, healthcare use and expenditures have gradually increased. Due to changing demographics and rising healthcare costs, the United States government has emphasized the need for enhanced value evaluation in healthcare spending; hence, the United States has adopted various strategies to control rising healthcare expenditures [5,6], focusing on medication costs as a significant target for potential savings. Furthermore, pharmaceutical companies in the United States have been required to submit economic studies on the implications of introducing new drugs to the Food and Drug Administration (FDA) [7].

As value-based care becomes increasingly relevant in patient care, pharmacoeconomics continues to gain prominence within the clinical setting [8], yet the subject occupies an uncertain place within professional pharmacy programs [9–11]. Rascati and colleagues conducted a study examining the extent of pharmacoeconomics education provided during the 1996–1997 academic year [9]. Of the 79 schools surveyed, 63 (80%) provided pharmacoeconomics education at the BS and/or PharmD level. Subsequent surveys conducted in 2007 and 2013 found that, while pharmacoeconomics education is provided in nearly all United States pharmacy programs, there is variation in the topics covered and in teaching hours [10,11]. Given that these studies are dated, there is currently a lack of information regarding the content of pharmacoeconomics taught within the current PharmD curriculum in United States-based pharmacy programs. Meanwhile, accreditation bodies, educational councils, and professional pharmacy organizations have consistently promoted pharmacoeconomics education and knowledge within the curricula of United States-based pharmacy programs for several years. The 2016 Accreditation Council for Pharmacy Education (ACPE) outlined the required elements of the didactic PharmD curriculum, including the following description of pharmacoeconomics as the "application of economic principles and theories to the provision of cost-effective pharmacy products and services that optimize patient-care outcomes, particularly in situations where healthcare resources are limited" [12]. Since 2010, the North American Pharmacist Licensure Examination has consistently included pharmacoeconomics competency statements [10,13]. Previously, the International Society for Pharmacoeconomics and Outcomes Research (ISPOR) Educators' Toolkit Task Force provided valuable teaching resources for pharmacoeconomics educators. In 2020, ISPOR introduced the 'New Competencies Framework for Health Economics and Outcomes Research Professionals' [14], which serves as a guide for academic curricula, fellowships, and continuing-education programs and for the evaluation of candidates for health economics and outcomes research (HEOR) career opportunities.

The role of pharmacists has extended beyond medication distribution to promoting sound and cost-effective drug therapy, enhancing patient outcomes, and contributing to the overall improvement of healthcare in the community [15–18]. Specifically, with pharmacists' knowledge of pharmacology, disease, anatomy, drug calculations, dosage, and drug–drug interactions, integrating pharmacoeconomics knowledge enables them to make informed therapeutic decisions. The acquisition of knowledge in pharmacoeconomics should allow pharmacists to assess and compare clinical guidelines, evaluate drug therapy recommendations, review data from clinical trials, and assess the economic impact of medications [16]. Hence, the potential role of pharmacists in integrating pharmacoeconomics into clinical practice is paramount [19]. As the healthcare industry experiences continuous innovation, the responsibilities of pharmacists and their role as pharmacoeconomics experts are also impacted, affecting the skillset required to adapt to the changing environment. Pharmacy programs must address the increasingly complex and specialized skills that employers desire. This study aims to assess the extent to which accredited pharmacy colleges in the United States cover pharmacoeconomics content within the didactic curricula of their Doctor of Pharmacy (PharmD) programs.

2. Materials and Methods

We systematically searched the curriculum websites of all 141 United States-based pharmacy programs holding accredited (full or candidate status) professional-degree programs to identify relevant pharmacoeconomics content. Information regarding pharmacoeconomics-related course descriptions, the number of credit hours, and syllabus content (if available) were determined for each pharmacy program and abstracted into a database. The data collection excluded graduate, post-doctoral, and fellowship-training programs, as the study focused exclusively on the PharmD degree. Our search did not cover elective courses or syllabi from experiential rotations because our assessment strictly focuses on required courses in the core curriculum. The location of the pharmacy programs was regionally classified based on four geographic regions established by the United States Census Bureau: the Northeast, Midwest, South, and West. Microsoft Excel for Microsoft 365 (Version 2310) was used to analyze the data [20].

Our study qualifies as a literature review and does not involve human subjects; thus, it does not require ethical or Institutional Review Board approval.

3. Results

Out of the 141 pharmacy programs included in the analysis, publicly available information on pharmacoeconomics content was identified on the websites of 111 programs. The relevant data from these programs were compiled in an Excel database, alphabetically listed for ease of reference. Of the included pharmacy programs, 57 (51%) were public institutions; 54 (49%) were private (Figure 1). Geographically, most of the assessed programs, 41 (37%), were in the South region. Notably, six of the pharmacy programs offered distance pathways or online PharmD education options.

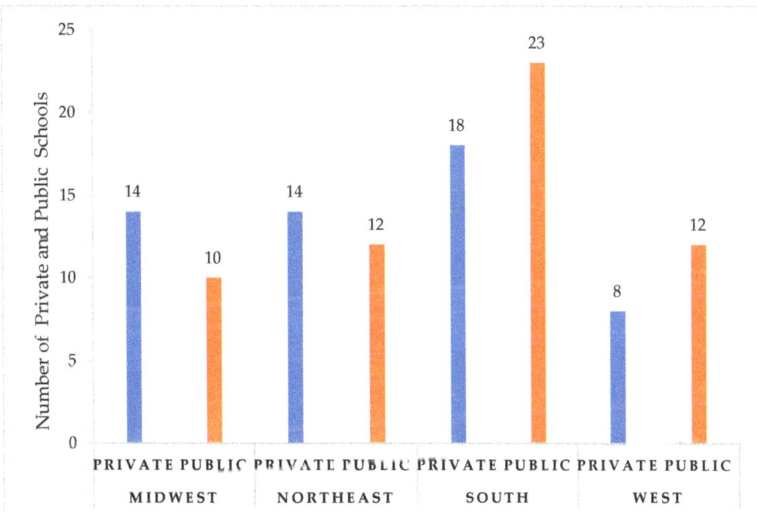

Figure 1. Distribution of assessed private and public pharmacy programs by region.

While some information regarding the curriculum was publicly accessible, a smaller proportion of pharmacy programs made their syllabi available online. Out of the 111 schools assessed, only 30 syllabi were retrieved from online sources. It is noteworthy, however, that all the pharmacy programs included in our database required the inclusion of pharmacoeconomics content within their curricula. Figure 2 shows that pharmacoeconomics teaching predominantly occurred during the third professional year (n = 55; 51%) and the second professional year (n = 39; 36%). All the required pharmacoeconomics courses exhibited similarities in terms of their learning objectives. A comprehensive list of these learning objectives is outlined as follows:

1. Define pharmacoeconomics;

2. Identify and determine the relevant costs and consequences associated with pharmacy products and services;
3. Define the differences between cost-benefit analysis (CBA), cost-effectiveness analysis (CEA), cost-minimization analysis (CMA), and cost-utility analysis (CUA);
4. Discuss the significance of specifying/selecting perspectives for inclusion in the analysis
5. Overview the steps involved in conducting a pharmacoeconomic analysis;
6. Critically evaluate current pharmacoeconomics literature;
7. Identify the potential applications of pharmacoeconomics in various pharmacy settings

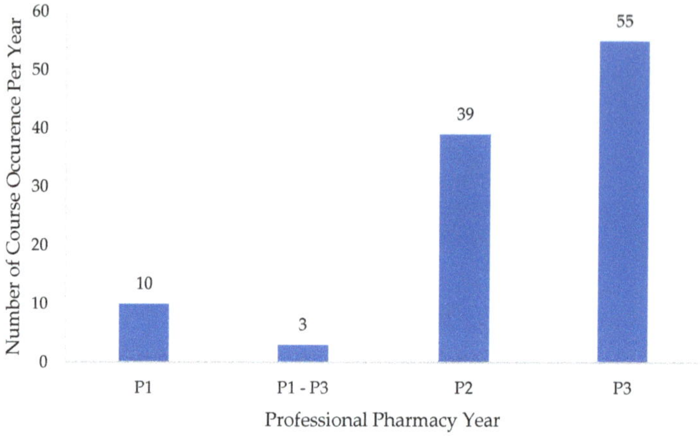

Figure 2. Pharmacoeconomics course occurrence by professional year (n = 107).

Course descriptions across the analyzed syllabi were generally broad and primarily focused on equipping students with introductory concepts or the principles of pharmacoeconomics. Nonetheless, there is a comprehensive consensus among several course descriptions that balancing the cost with the consequences (outcomes) of pharmaceutical therapies and services is the overarching goal of pharmacoeconomics in PharmD education.

Figure 3 shows that the number of credit hours allocated to pharmacoeconomics education varied from one to seven. The majority of programs assigned either two credit hours (n = 54) or three credit hours (n = 45) to pharmacoeconomics topics; yet it is worth highlighting that those credit hours are not exclusive to pharmacoeconomics and are distributed among several topics integrated within one course. The amount and nature of the delivery of pharmacoeconomics or pharmacoeconomics-related content vary between programs. While most programs offered a required core course solely focused on pharmacoeconomics, others incorporated pharmacoeconomics alongside related subjects such as pharmacoepidemiology, population health, and pharmacy administration. Additionally, in some programs, pharmacoeconomics content was covered within a broader course encompassing various topics, including pharmacokinetics, pharmacodynamics, pharmacoepidemiology, and pharmacotherapy related to patient care.

The identified pharmacoeconomics topics were referenced within course descriptions, and the syllabi were categorized and presented based on 20 emerging topics, arranged in alphabetical order in Table 1. The majority of syllabi from the reviewed programs covered various methods of pharmacoeconomics analysis, although only about half (n = 54; 49%) of the reviewed programs' syllabi mentioned the application of pharmacoeconomics. There were various ways to foster and assess students' learning outcomes in the pharmacoeconomics course. Teaching methods varied and encompassed didactic lectures, guest speakers, videos, research projects, problem-based learning, case studies, and article-critiquing assignments. Notably, based on the information analyzed, no program that taught pharmacoeconomics in an interdisciplinary setting was identified. Reading assignments were prevalent in the reviewed syllabi, while several featured unique assignments designed to foster student engagement, ownership of learning, and productive interactions among peers. Such assignments included research projects, presentations, and group work. In the reviewed syllabi, skills were not identified as a significant part of the descriptions and objectives of the pharmacoeconomics courses.

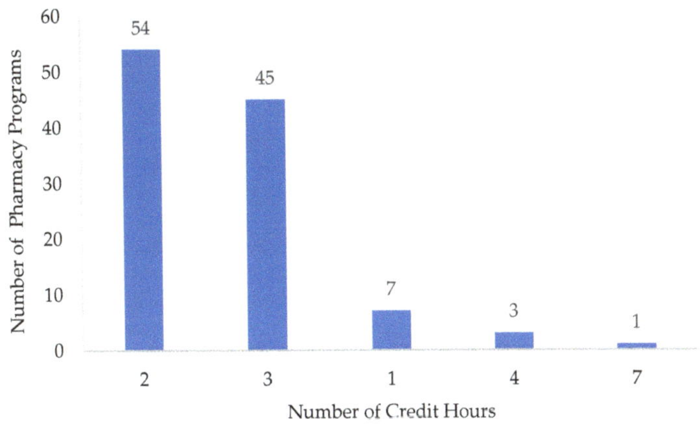

Figure 3. Semester credit hour distribution for pharmacoeconomics (n = 110).

Table 1. Common topics covered in pharmacoeconomics courses.

1. Costs
2. Cost-benefit analysis (CBA)
3. Cost-effectiveness analysis (CEA)
4. Cost-minimization analysis (CMA)
5. Cost of illness (COI)
6. Cost-utility analysis (CUA)
7. Disability-adjusted life year (DALY)
8. Decision analysis
9. Effectiveness
10. Efficacy
11. Health-related quality of life (HRQOL)
12. Health technology assessment (HTA)
13. Markov model
14. Patient-reported outcomes (PROs)
15. Quality-adjusted life year (QALY)
16. Sensitivity analysis
17. Systematic review
18. Utility
19. Value-based pricing (VBP)
20. Willingness to pay (WTP)

As the sub-discipline of pharmacoeconomics has advanced, an extensive array of textbooks has become accessible. However, it is worth noting that many excellent pharmacoeconomics books authored outside the United States are inevitably shaped by the unique healthcare funding and provision systems of their respective countries. Consequently, their focus may not always align with the primary concerns and issues encountered in the United States healthcare system. Most pharmacoeconomics courses (n = 68; 61%) did not explicitly require a textbook. The courses that did require one were mostly assigned "Essentials of Pharmacoeconomics" by Karen Rascati [2]. Other courses assigned pharmacoeconomics chapter readings from other books related to pharmacy research, pharmacoepidemiology, and drug literature evaluation. Most of these readings are available through comprehensive online pharmacy resources, which several pharmacy schools subscribe to. Other readings consisted of reports, journal articles, and handouts, which were utilized to provide real-world pharmacoeconomics applications and to reinforce key concepts.

4. Discussion

A comprehensive literature search uncovered only three studies evaluating application-based or active learning in a pharmacoeconomics course within the United States PharmD curriculum [21–23]. Our evaluation of pharmacoeconomics curricula and instructional methods revealed a shift towards incorporating more active learning approaches; however, the impact of this shift has yet to be assessed. There are no resources or reports specifying the expectations of employers regarding pharmacoeconomics competencies in new PharmD graduates. Based on our professional assessment of the course syllabus, the skills provided were primarily foundational, especially considering the growing momentum surrounding pharmacoeconomics methods. Those foundational skills consist primarily of identifying the determinants of the health economy, different types of pharmacoeconomics evaluations, and critically analyzing pharmacoeconomics and outcome literature. To equip students with advanced-level skills, pharmacy programs should consider providing technical resources and training opportunities that emphasize practical application. Such advanced-level skills enable students to conduct trial- and modeling-based economic evaluations and indirect treatment comparisons, perform calculations involved in decision analysis, and engage in risk adjustment and Markov modeling.

The learning modality of pharmacoeconomics should encompass a combination of didactic training, laboratory training, and experiential learning [22–24]. Experiential learning is of particular importance as it is one of the most effective ways to enhance pharmacoeconomics education by engaging students through active learning strategies and fostering collaborations with industry exposure. Active learning sessions incorporate problem-solving exercises, case discussions, and laboratory activities. By actively participating in laboratory work, pharmacy students can develop a deeper understanding of the overall process involved in conducting pharmacoeconomics evaluation, as outlined by Jolicoeur and colleagues, which consists of ten steps: (1) defining the problem, (2) determining the study's perspective, (3) determining the alternatives and outcomes, (4) selecting the appropriate pharmacoeconomics method, (5) placing monetary values on the outcomes, (6) identifying study resources, (7) establishing the probabilities of the outcomes, (8) applying decision analysis, (9) discounting costs or performing a sensitivity or incremental cost analysis, and (10) presenting the results, along with any limitations of the study [25]. Through these laboratory activities, students could learn how the results of pharmacoeconomics evaluations are translated and applied in clinical practice to support decisions in various areas, including individual patient treatment, disease management, drug-use guideline development, and formulary management. Additionally, pharmacy programs can significantly benefit from establishing educational partnerships with the industry. These partnerships can take the form of practical experiences or internships, providing students with valuable industry exposure, bridging the gap between classroom learning and real-world job experience, and equipping them with advanced skills and the knowledge necessary for successful careers in pharmacoeconomics.

Pharmacy education standards in the United States have undergone a substantial transformation, expanding beyond conventional basic science and clinical subjects. In light of recent developments in pharmacy education and the continuous implementation of curricular redesigns across these programs, [26–28], educators must formulate curricular strategies that are in harmony with the emerging trends in the field, which encompass aspects of pharmacoeconomics. The availability of data and information concerning pharmacoeconomics education in United States pharmacy programs is limited and needs to be updated. To accurately assess the current state of pharmacoeconomics education, our study examined the curriculum content of all accredited pharmacy programs in the United States, focusing on three key areas: course description, number of credit hours, and syllabus content (if available). Specifically, the assessment focused on core required courses rather than electives or experiential training, aiming to determine the extent to which all pharmacy students were exposed to pharmacoeconomics content during their PharmD program. The data we gathered reveal significant variations in the offerings of pharmacoeconomics programs within the PharmD curriculum, including variations in the number of credit hours, teaching hours, and the specific year in which the teaching occurred.

While pharmacoeconomics has been incorporated as a compulsory or elective course in schools or colleges of pharmacy in many countries, the variation observed in pharmacoeconomics education in the United States has also been noted globally [29,30]. A literature review examining the global trend of pharmacoeconomics courses in undergraduate pharmacy education revealed significant variability in course content [29]. Similarly, a study focusing on Eastern Mediterranean region pharmacy schools found a wide range of classroom hours dedicated to required courses covering pharmacoeconomics-related topics, varying from 2 to 60 hours among the different schools [30]. The fact that pharmacoeconomics instruction primarily occurs in the later stages of the didactic curriculum may provide students with the necessary problem-solving skills to apply pharmacoeconomics principles in clinical practice and guide clinical and policy decision-making. Since pharmacoeconomics goes beyond the economic evaluation of medical programs and pharmaceutical drugs, encompassing recommendations for efficiently utilizing healthcare resources, pharmacoeconomics knowledge must be reinforced through advanced pharmacy practice experiences or clinical rotations. Furthermore, because pharmacoeconomics takes a scientific approach to comparing the value of pharmaceutical products and services, its teaching has the potential to address various issues associated with drug affordability, such as drug access, medication adherence, patient outcomes, and health disparities.

Educational research within the pharmacy field has consistently demonstrated that evidence-based teaching and learning strategies positively impact student learning outcomes [31–33]. The fact that there is a lack of scholarship in teaching and learning (SoTL) focusing on pharmacoeconomics raises some questions about the priority given to this topic in pharmacy education. Engaging in SoTL focused on pharmacoeconomics can lead to evidence-based improvements in teaching practices, curriculum development, and student learning outcomes in this discipline. These efforts can also foster a culture of continuous improvement and innovation in pharmacoeconomics education in the PharmD curriculum. As the adoption of evidence-based instructional strategies becomes more widespread in pharmacy classrooms and practice, it becomes increasingly important to focus on the teaching and learning of pharmacoeconomics. Furthermore, there needs to be more sufficient data on PharmD students' perceptions, motivations, and attitudes toward pharmacoeconomics in the United States. This highlights the need for pharmacy educators to make increased efforts to assess the impact of students' behavior and their learning experiences related to pharmacoeconomics. By examining these factors, educators can gain valuable insights and further enhance the teaching and learning of pharmacoeconomics to meet pharmacy students' needs effectively.

To the best of our knowledge, this is the only recent work that has investigated the state of pharmacoeconomics education in the United States regarding course objectives, number of credit hours, and syllabus content. However, our assessment does have some limitations worth acknowledging. First, several pharmacy programs did not publicly have their curriculum information posted on their main website, preventing us from assessing those programs. We did not contact the school representatives of such programs to obtain information regarding aspects of their curricula that were not accessible online. Second, our search methodology focused solely on identifying pharmacoeconomics-related content, meaning we may have missed other courses that cover concepts related to pharmacoeconomics but do not explicitly mention them. It is important to consider these limitations when interpreting the findings of our study. Future research could explore additional sources or methods to gather comprehensive data on pharmacoeconomics education in the United States, addressing these limitations and providing a more comprehensive understanding of the current state of pharmacoeconomics education. In future investigations, it would be crucial to longitudinally assess student learning and retention within the realm of pharmacoeconomics.

5. Proposed Recommendations

Taken individually, the results of this review lack the conclusive evidence needed to guide the comprehensive development or revision of a detailed plan for thoroughly integrating pharmacoeconomics into a pharmacy curriculum. Nonetheless, the results do point to essential principles that should be considered when educating pharmacy students to actively engage with pharmacoeconomics. They are as follows:

- The extensive implementation of problem-based learning in pharmacy schools offers a valuable opportunity for the seamless integration of pharmacoeconomics education across the curriculum. This integration will allow students to appreciate the subject's significance in clinical practice and its fundamental role in shaping healthcare decision-making.
- Teaching needs to ensure that pharmacy students appreciate the relevance of learning the skills required to critically evaluate the effect of different healthcare interventions on patients. One way to accomplish this task is to introduce the concepts related to pharmacoeconomics early in the pharmacy curriculum and to build on and reinforce these concepts throughout the rest of the curriculum. The literature suggests that early one-off training is linked with poor knowledge in the long term [34,35]. When students are introduced to pharmacoeconomics and acquire related skills during their early years of PharmD education but do not continue to engage with this topic throughout the remainder of their training, they not only lose the acquired knowledge and skills but also any sense of their relevance.
- Reinforce pharmacoeconomics knowledge with relevant, real-world examples from peer-reviewed articles on topics of interest to students. For instance, learning about an incremental cost-effectiveness ratio could be embedded within consideration of a peer-reviewed article reporting the results of a clinical trial of combination antiretroviral therapy for human immunodeficiency virus.
- Patient cases spanning a diverse range of medical conditions across various practice settings could incorporate pharmacoeconomics principles. This integration challenges students to adopt a comprehensive perspective, considering not only the presented medical condition but also the pharmacoeconomics evidence underpinning treatment decisions.
- Illustrate how pharmacoeconomics and related knowledge/skills are used in daily pharmacy practice. Examples can be designed to demonstrate that pharmacoeconomics data can inform formulary decisions, aid in the selection or removal of drugs, and guide the development of practice guidelines aimed at promoting the cost-effective and appropriate utilization of pharmaceutical products. Other examples can explain that, in a community pharmacy setting, pharmacoeconomics can be applied by conducting a cost-effectiveness analysis of two common medications used to manage a chronic condition like hypertension. By comparing the total costs and health outcomes associated with Drug A and Drug B over a specified period, pharmacists can provide evidence-based recommendations to patients and healthcare providers, helping them make informed decisions about the most cost-effective treatment option while ensuring optimal health outcomes and resource utilization.
- Use of journal clubs in pharmacoeconomics education. Journal clubs are indispensable assets in pharmacoeconomics education for several fundamental reasons. To begin with, they serve as catalysts for critical thinking by necessitating students to dissect and appraise pharmacoeconomics research articles, thereby refining students' capacity to scrutinize evidence and make well-informed decisions in clinical practice. Second, they act as a mechanism to ensure that students continuously stay abreast of the swiftly evolving realm of pharmacoeconomics, nurturing a culture of lifelong learning.

Third, these clubs elevate communication proficiencies, empowering students to proficiently elucidate intricate pharmacoeconomic concepts to peers and fellow healthcare practitioners. Last, they foster collaboration and teamwork, which are indispensable competencies in healthcare environments that mandate interdisciplinary synergy for the provision of optimal patient care.

- Implement debates as a means to invigorate discussions on pharmacoeconomics subjects while acquiring proficiency in presentation techniques and critical assessment. A recent study demonstrated the efficacy of employing debates as an educational instrument, highlighting their capacity to augment students' critical thinking abilities and aptitude for appraising pharmacoeconomics literature [36]. Moreover, the study reveals that this approach elevates students' self-assurance in decision-making, enhances their critical analysis of evidence, and refines their communication skills for articulating arguments effectively.
- Students can gain advanced pharmacoeconomics knowledge and skills through comprehensive research projects offered within elective courses, capstone experiences, or summer research internships. These student-led research initiatives offer a unique opportunity for students to deepen their understanding of pharmacoeconomics, effectively connecting theoretical concepts to practical applications. These immersive experiences equip students with essential skills in data analysis, modeling, and the critical evaluation of healthcare interventions, making them well prepared for future challenges in the field.
- PharmD students aiming to acquire advanced pharmacoeconomics training beyond the standard didactic curriculum should have the opportunity to enroll in an advanced pharmacoeconomics elective. Typically, these electives are standalone courses that expand upon the foundational pharmacoeconomics curriculum. While introductory courses introduce students to fundamental pharmacoeconomics analysis methods, advanced pharmacoeconomics electives delve deeper, covering complex topics like multiple criteria decision analysis, discrete event simulations, Bayesian analysis, machine learning methods, artificial intelligence, value-based pricing, and health technology assessment. Through hands-on projects and case studies, students gain practical experience in conducting pharmacoeconomics evaluations, interpreting results, and effectively communicating their findings to stakeholders. These advanced courses equip future pharmacists with the research skills necessary to navigate the dynamic pharmaceutical industry and make substantial contributions to evidence-based practice.
- Tailor the instruction to a suitable level for students, acknowledging the wide-ranging educational backgrounds and experiences of PharmD students. Consider offering specialized tutoring sessions for students seeking extra support to ensure comprehensive support for all students.
- Pharmacoeconomics requires regular educational material updates for several crucial reasons. First, healthcare landscapes evolve rapidly, with new medications, technologies, and treatment approaches emerging frequently. Staying current ensures that students and professionals can apply the latest methodologies and data for accurate analysis and decision-making. Second, economic factors, such as inflation and changing healthcare policies, affect cost assessments and pricing strategies, necessitating adjustments in educational content. Moreover, updating materials fosters continuous learning and adaptability, enhancing the competency of practitioners in optimizing healthcare resource allocation and improving patient outcomes, ultimately reflecting the dynamic nature of pharmacoeconomics in modern healthcare.
- Establishing partnerships between academia and industry presents an opportunity to advance pharmacoeconomics knowledge within an academic context. Strategies like internships, industry mentors, on-site visits, and collaborative projects utilizing shared data are promising initiatives in this regard.

6. Conclusions

Training in pharmacoeconomics can be valuable for any healthcare professional who engages with patients and their families or communities. To understand the status of pharmacoeconomics education in professional pharmacy programs within the United States, we reviewed catalogs of 111 pharmacy programs. Despite the recognized importance of pharmacoeconomics in evidence-based care and drug-prescribing processes, our findings indicate uncertainty regarding the extent to which all pharmacy programs across the United States dedicate adequate credit hours to balance both the theoretical and practical considerations of pharmacoeconomics in their curricula. The pharmacy profession is quickly evolving, and today, pharmacists practice not only in traditional settings such as community pharmacies and hospitals but also in other settings requiring pharmacoeconomics knowledge. This requires pharmacy programs that plan to prepare today's pharmacy students to meet tomorrow's healthcare challenges by finding the appropriate balance between pharmacoeconomics course content, contact hours, and delivery methods that can meet the needs of students in realizing their future career goals.

Author Contributions: Conceptualization, G.A.; methodology, G.A.; software, G.A. and S.A.Y.A.; formal analysis, G.A., J.S. and C.S.C.; investigation, G.A.; data curation, G.A., J.S. and C.S.C.; writing—original draft preparation, G.A., S.A.Y.A., A.A.A., J.S. and C.S.C.; writing—review and editing, G.A., S.A.Y.A., A.A.A., J.S. and C.S.C.; visualization, G.A. and S.A.Y.A.; supervision, G.A.; project administration, G.A. All authors have read and agreed to the published version of the manuscript.

Funding: This research received no external funding.

Institutional Review Board Statement: Not applicable.

Informed Consent Statement: Not applicable.

Data Availability Statement: The data presented in this study are available upon request from the corresponding author.

Conflicts of Interest: The authors declare no conflict of interest.

References

1. Mauskopf, J.A. Why study pharmacoeconomics? *Expert Rev. Pharmacoecon. Outcomes Res.* **2001**, *1*, 1–3. [CrossRef] [PubMed]
2. Rascati, K. *Essentials of Pharmacoeconomics*; Lippincott Williams & Wilkins: Philadelphia, PA, USA, 2013; p. 3.
3. Patel, V.; Shah, M. Artificial intelligence and machine learning in drug discovery and development. *Intell. Med.* **2022**, *2*, 134–140. [CrossRef]
4. Prendergast, M.E.; Burdick, J.A. Recent advances in enabling technologies in 3D printing for precision medicine. *Adv. Mater.* **2020**, *32*, 1902516. [CrossRef] [PubMed]
5. Ikeda, S.; Ikegami, N.; Oliver, A.J.; Ikeda, M. A case for the adoption of pharmacoeconomic guidelines in Japan. *PharmacoEconomics* **1996**, *10*, 546–551. [CrossRef]
6. Chiang, P.J.; Einarson, T. A survey of pharmacoeconomics in the Canadian pharmaceutical industry. *Drug Inf. J.* **1998**, *32*, 619–627. [CrossRef]
7. Niyazov, A.; Lenci, D. Communicating healthcare economic and pre-approval information with healthcare decision-makers: Opportunities following the 21st century cures act and FDA guidance. *Front. Public Health* **2018**, *6*, 304. [CrossRef]
8. Kamae, I. Value-based approaches to healthcare systems and pharmacoeconomics requirements in Asia: South Korea, Taiwan, Thailand and Japan. *PharmacoEconomics* **2010**, *28*, 831–838. [CrossRef]
9. Rascati, K.; Therese, C.M.; Draugalis, J.R. Pharmacoeconomic education in US schools of pharmacy. *Am. J. Pharm. Educ.* **1998**, *62*, 167.
10. Makhinova, T.; Rascati, K. Pharmacoeconomics education in US colleges and schools of pharmacy. *Am. J. Pharm. Educ.* **2013**, *77*, 145. [CrossRef]
11. Reddy, M.; Rascati, K.; Wahawisan, J.; Rascati, M. Pharmacoeconomic education in US colleges and schools of pharmacy: An update. *Am. J. Pharm. Educ.* **2008**, *72*, 51. [CrossRef]
12. Accreditation Council for Pharmacy Education. *Education. Accreditation Standards and Key Elements for the Professional Program in Pharmacy Leading to the Doctor of Pharmacy Degree ("Standards 2016")*; Accreditation Council for Pharmacy Education: Chicago, IL, USA, 2017.
13. National Association of Boards Pharmacy. North American Pharmacist Licensure Examination®(NAPLEX®) Competency Statements (As of January 2021). Available online: https://nabp.pharmacy/programs/examinations/naplex/competency-statements-2021/ (accessed on 30 May 2023).

14. Pizzi, L.T.; Onukwugha, E.; Corey, R.; Albarmawi, H.; Murray, J. Competencies for Professionals in Health Economics and Outcomes Research: The ISPOR Health Economics and Outcomes Research Competencies Framework. *Value Health* **2020**, *23*, 1120–1127. [CrossRef] [PubMed]
15. Goode, J.-V.; Owen, J.; Page, A.; Gatewood, S. Community-based pharmacy practice innovation and the role of the community-based pharmacist practitioner in the United States. *Pharmacy* **2019**, *7*, 106. [CrossRef] [PubMed]
16. Dalton, K.; Byrne, S. Role of the pharmacist in reducing healthcare costs: Current insights. *Integr. Pharm. Res. Pract.* **2017**, *6*, 37. [CrossRef] [PubMed]
17. Compton, W.M.; Jones, C.M.; Stein, J.B.; Wargo, E.M. Promising roles for pharmacists in addressing the US opioid crisis. *Res. Soc. Adm. Pharm.* **2019**, *15*, 910–916. [CrossRef] [PubMed]
18. Reeves, L.; Robinson, K.; McClelland, T.; Adedoyin, C.A.; Broeseker, A.; Adunlin, G. Pharmacist interventions in the management of blood pressure control and adherence to antihypertensive medications: A systematic review of randomized controlled trials. *J. Pharm. Pract.* **2021**, *34*, 480–492. [CrossRef]
19. Farid, S.; Baines, D. Pharmacoeconomics Education in the Middle East and North Africa Region: A Web-Based Research Project. *Value Health Reg. Issues* **2021**, *25*, 182–188. [CrossRef]
20. Microsoft Corporation. Microsoft Excel. 2023. Available online: https://office.microsoft.com/excel (accessed on 13 April 2020).
21. Stewart, D.W.; Brown, S.D.; Clavier, C.W.; Wyatt, J. Active-learning processes used in US pharmacy education. *Am. J. Pharm. Educ.* **2011**, *75*, 68. [CrossRef]
22. Frederick, K.D.; Havrda, D.E.; Scott, D.; Gatwood, J.; Hall, E.A.; Desselle, S.P.; Hohmeier, K.C. Assessing Student Perceptions of Blended and Online Learning Courses in Pharmacoeconomics, Management, and Leadership. *Am. J. Pharm. Educ.* **2023**, *87*, ajpe9001. [CrossRef]
23. Edwards, A.; Oestreich, J.H. A novel game to review pharmacoeconomic content in a pharmacy program. *Curr. Pharm. Teach. Learn.* **2022**, *14*, 1193–1198. [CrossRef]
24. Shih, Y.-C.T.; Kauf, T.L.; Biddle, A.L.; Simpson, K.N. Incorporating problem-based learning concepts into a lecture-based pharmacoeconomics course. *Am. J. Pharm. Educ.* **1999**, *63*, 152–159.
25. Jolicoeur, L.M.; Jones-Grizzle, A.J.; Boyer, J.G. Guidelines for performing a pharmacoeconomic analysis. *Am. J. Hosp. Pharm.* **1992**, *49*, 1741–1747. [CrossRef] [PubMed]
26. Bzowyckyj, A.; Bradley, B.; Cawley, P.; Nuziale, B.; White, S. Adapting a National Framework to Inform Curricular Redesign Focused on Enhancing Student Clinical Competency. *Pharmacy* **2021**, *9*, 89. [CrossRef] [PubMed]
27. Wright, B.M.; Hornsby, L.; Marlowe, K.F.; Fowlin, J.; Surry, D.W. Innovating pharmacy curriculum through backward design. *TechTrends* **2018**, *62*, 224–229. [CrossRef]
28. Rhoney, D.H.; Singleton, S.; Nelson, N.R.; Anderson, S.M.; Hubal, R. Forces driving change in pharmacy education: Opportunities to take academic, social, technological, economic, and political into the future. *J. Am. Coll. Clin. Pharm.* **2021**, *4*, 639–651. [CrossRef]
29. Thomas, D.; Sundararaj, K.G.S.; Shirwaikar, A.; Tarn, Y.H. Inclusion of pharmacoeconomics course in the undergraduate pharmacy education: A global trend review. *Indian J. Pharm. Pract.* **2016**, *9*, 147–151. [CrossRef]
30. Alefan, Q.; AlImam, S.; Mukattash, T.; Mhaidat, N.; Alabbadi, I.; Rascati, K. Pharmacoeconomics education in WHO Eastern Mediterranean region. *Curr. Pharm. Teach. Learn.* **2015**, *7*, 819–825. [CrossRef]
31. Gleason, B.L.; Peeters, M.J.; Resman-Targoff, B.H.; Karr, S.; McBane, S.; Kelley, K.; Thomas, T.; Denetclaw, T.H. An active-learning strategies primer for achieving ability-based educational outcomes. *Am. J. Pharm. Educ.* **2011**, *75*, 186. [CrossRef]
32. Aburahma, M.H.; Mohamed, H.M. Educational games as a teaching tool in pharmacy curriculum. *Am. J. Pharm. Educ.* **2015**, *79*, 59. [CrossRef]
33. Franks, A.M.; Payakachat, N. Positioning the scholarship of teaching and learning squarely on the center of the desk. *Am. J. Pharm. Educ.* **2020**, *84*, ajpe8046. [CrossRef]
34. Hailikari, T.; Katajavuori, N.; Lindblom-Ylanne, S. The relevance of prior knowledge in learning and instructional design. *Am. J. Pharm. Educ.* **2008**, *72*, 113. [CrossRef]
35. Nathanson, C.; Paulhus, D.L.; Williams, K.M. The challenge to cumulative learning: Do introductory courses actually benefit advanced students? *Teach. Psychol.* **2004**, *31*, 5–9. [CrossRef]
36. Alaqeel, S.; Alghamdi, A.; Balkhi, B.; Almazrou, S.; Alaujan, S. Impact of using debates in a pharmacoeconomic course on students' self-reported perceptions of skills acquired. *Pharm. Educ.* **2021**, *21*, 276–282. [CrossRef]

MDPI
St. Alban-Anlage 66
4052 Basel
Switzerland
www.mdpi.com

Healthcare Editorial Office
E-mail: healthcare@mdpi.com
www.mdpi.com/journal/healthcare